nourish *eat* repeat

Janelle,
Nourish, Eat,
and Enjoy!
-Arianne

nourish
eat
repeat

a busy woman's guide
to a healthier mind, body, and life

Adrianne Delgado, RD, LDN

Cover photo by Crystal Weise
Cover and interior design by Cathy Duffy

Printed in the United States of America

To Lucretia Page,
For always believing in this project and me.

table of contents

forward

by Jim Delgado

Let me paint a picture of the typical school day in 2019 with our family of seven. Our oldest of five children just got on the early bus; phase one is complete. The other four are beginning to stir. The more kids you have, the greater the risk that one or more of them will have a bad morning or will insist on sleeping just a little longer.

After three to four "this is the last time" warnings, one or two of them starts to make their way into the kitchen to eat. Nothing can prepare you for this! The feeding frenzy and insanity picks up momentum: dishes start to pile up in the sink, the refrigerator alarm lets us know the door has been left open, and the intermittent teasing is initiated. The kids start packing their lunch bags only to realize yesterday's empty containers and ice packs were never removed. Time ticks on, the second bus is coming shortly, and teeth still need to be brushed. Water bottles are packed, but three of them have not eaten yet.

Okay ... the second oldest has left on the bus and phase two is over. The final phase begins with only three kids to go and 10 minutes left on the clock. The final minute comes quickly and so does the familiar sound of "where are my shoes?" When the last three walk down the driveway to get the bus, the bus driver pulls up and comments about our "perfect family." We politely smile as we sigh with relief. Does this count for today's cardio workout? My beating heart says yes.

This is a fairly typical start to a day in the life of my wife, Adrianne Delgado, and me. In the middle of all this (the school, home, and workday responsibilities), Adrianne decided to write a book about food, family, and the "fun" surrounding it all, including the craziness!

Adrianne initially went to school to be a doctor, but quickly realized the profession was not compatible with the large family of which she always dreamed. After a few course changes, the world of food and nutrition became her focus and where she chose to dedicate her time and energy.

She went on to graduate with honors from West Chester University where she received a Bachelor's degree in nutrition and a minor in psychology. Both educational specialties have come in handy on a regular basis at home and at work. I am still not sure which environment requires the use of both areas of study more. Amidst the time spent studying, she somehow managed to find time to be the top-ranked women's tennis player at West Chester.

Food is a relaxing thought. It smells good, looks good, and tastes good. For many of us, food and mealtime play an important role in our lives. This book will take you on a unique journey to enhance your daily experience. It is a collection of human interaction—personal and practical advice—with enlightening revelations.

Whether it is the latest diet craze, giving in to the powerful marketing of food and restaurants, or the struggle with time restraints to slow down and eat quality food with those we care about most; many of us struggle in our relationship with food throughout our lives. This original reading will use the shared experiences and stories of others, and personal trials and tributes, combined with professional direction on how to work your way through the common struggles and misconceptions related to food.

Adrianne is the author of this real-life journey. Through her personal experiences, it has shaped her outlook, helped her understanding, and ultimately provided her with problem-solving skills. Somehow, Adrianne has found the motivation to take on the many challenges in her life, balancing a business, home and work responsibilities, church, the demands of a large family, and friends.

Healthy eating does not have to be so difficult. Without traditional "dieting"—which we all know has limited results—but through education, we can achieve this better way of life in a pleasurable and easy way.

We often say "life happens," but when we have a plan, we are better prepared to adapt and overcome. In the pages that follow, you will encounter engaging stories, relatable examples, and commonsense guidelines for cooking and eating, and they will also encourage each of us to simply choose to live a better life with those we care about most.

Excuses and unlikely scenarios are what Adrianne hears on a daily basis in the office setting of BodyMetrix, but those things are definitely not what she uses to combat her own challenges in life. That is not to say she doesn't have days that are tougher than others. She definitely does have her share, as do each of us. Striving to be a leader in all aspects of her life, she educates through example with compassion, commitment, and accountability—to her faith, her patients, her family and friends, and to herself. I believe this is what motivates her to succeed and why she strives to bring those in her life on this path.

What we all desire for our families and ourselves is a good, long, healthy life, and this book will help clarify what we should be eating, why we should be eating it, and how we should go about doing so. Through this collaboration of short stories, she hopes to help you "set the table" for success with food for you and for your family, all while balancing the many demands of today's busy world.

Enjoy, bon appetite!

introduction

There are two instances that stick out in particular when it comes to my childhood and being weight focused. The first was in fifth grade when I started noticing I was larger than my peers. I wouldn't call my younger self obese, but I was definitely chunky, which is totally normal for pre-pubescent girls. Instead of playing kickball or foursquare out at recess with the rest of the kids, I was trying to convince my friends to join my aerobics class out in the yard. The second instance was when I was in middle school and visiting my grandparents over the summer. My grandmother was known to speak her mind and that was one of my favorite things about her. I guarantee you, if she was still living, she would have no recollection of this conversation, but I remember it like it was yesterday.

"You have legs like your dad and his legs are fat," she said to me one day that summer.

Words have such an amazing impact on what we believe about ourselves. This particular statement held a lot of weight, no pun intended.

I do need to be clear that my parents never once commented about my weight or my food choices. I was allowed to eat pretty much anything I wanted, consuming both healthy and not-so-healthy foods. Well, anything except Fruit Rollups. My mom was a hard "no" when it came to those.

I had decent self-confidence, had several close friends, and earned good grades in school. I had a great childhood, yet there was also this part of me that felt like I wasn't good enough. I wish I hadn't focused so much on the negatives, but I have to believe it molded me into who I am today.

My personal struggles have created a level of empathy within and a desire to help others, which is why I'm good at my job. The thorn in my side, if you will, is always trying to get out of my own head, but it's also what grounds me. It allows me to rely on Jesus instead of my own pride. I honestly think if I got all of this nutrition thing right all of the time, I would become self-reliant, prideful, and boastful—three things that scare the living daylights out of me. If nothing else, you can always count on my honesty, even if it exposes my vulnerability. I have found that bringing both honesty and vulnerability to the surface creates a space for healing.

As I'm writing this, I am 39 years old. I grew up in Lancaster County in a quiet rural area. Contrary to what non-native Pennsylvanians think, not everyone from Lancaster County is Amish—nor am I. In high school, I enjoyed playing sports and eventually went on to play tennis for my college.

I met my husband on a blind date set up by his sister, Brenda. Our first date didn't go that well, but thankfully, the story ended happily. Brenda and I were in the same Bible study group in college. One evening, she showed me a picture of her brother and asked if I would consider going out on a date with him since she thought we had a lot in common. I hadn't dated anyone for a couple months, so I was interested in meeting someone new. We decided to double date with Brenda and her boyfriend.

Looking back, I think Jim felt awkward with his little sister attending our date. We saw the movie *Remember the Titans* and then went out to eat at a local diner. As you know, movies aren't the best place to get to know a person better and by the end of the night we had barely spoken more than a couple sentences to each other. Since the diner was near my apartment, it made sense to drop me off first, which meant Jim and I had an audience to politely say our goodbyes.

I remember walking into my apartment and telling my roommates, "If he never calls again, that is completely okay with me." Funny enough, he did end up calling that night to apologize for not walking me to the door, noting it was awkward with his sister in the car, and we ended up having a great conversation.

A year later, we were engaged, and a year after that, we married. We have five kids—three boys and twin girls—and live on a farm that once belonged to Jim's grandparents. At one point, I had five children ages six and under. To say it was a circus would be an understatement.

On a particular trip to Kohl's, Jim had all five kids with him while I ran to the bathroom. When I walked up to my family, the kids were running around as Jim was frantically trying to corral them to one location. A woman passing by exclaimed, "Wow, you have five kids? How wonderful!" Before she could finish, Jim, anticipating the words we had heard countless times before, snapped back, "Yes, I get it … we are freaking blessed!"

Sometimes the stress of it all gets to us, but we always try to find the humor. We live in an old farmhouse, which means the rooms are small, there isn't much closet space, and all of the kids share rooms. There's no way to know who did what. Everyone's favorite line is, "It wasn't me!" Because of this, I frequently punish the wrong child.

There's no privacy. We all share a small bathroom. Every winter, we spend a small fortune on oil for heat since our stone walls are not well insulated. What we do have is a fairly large outdoor space where we spend most of our time playing and growing vegetables. When you have a large family, you need to save money somewhere. My friends often tease that my house is so out of character with the rest of the suburban landscape surrounding us.

There is no doubt in my mind that Jim and I are meant to be together. He is kind, he is a great father, and he loves me no matter what I throw at him. I can be dramatic and emotional at times (like only a female can) and he loves me anyway. He grounds me when I am emotional and supports every one of my dreams, no matter how crazy.

Jim is always thinking of others and he teaches me how to be more patient, forgiving, and thoughtful. He is calm and quiet when I'm loud and frazzled. I tend to make decisions quickly and he takes his time, which is good in some situations, but not at restaurants when it's time to order! We complement each other in so many ways and I'm so thankful he's in my life.

Jim loves nature and sports. He has taught our kids to be observant of both other people and the environment, which is a skill I sometimes lack, but am learning too. I know there are times we drive each other crazy, but at the end of the day, we are committed to our family, no matter what.

Together, we own a small health and wellness company called BodyMetrix, located in the middle of Limerick, Pennsylvania, which is a suburb that sits 45 minutes west of Philadelphia. I'm a registered dietitian by trade and he's a massage therapist with a degree in exercise physiology. We decided to pool our resources and create a business to provide a unique and comprehensive service for our clientele. Running a business together poses its own set of challenges, but there is no one else I trust more. Our common goal of helping others is what has made BodyMetrix the successful business it is today, and it is my hope that our patients sense warmth and genuineness when they walk through our door.

Needless to say, I stumbled on this journey of writing in a profoundly unique way. Sitting at breakfast one morning, I found myself trading stories with my girlfriends about all of the crazy adventures our families have encountered over the years. After the laughter died down from one particular story I told, my friend turned toward me, looked me in the eyes, and said, "You are writing all of this down somewhere, right?"

The thought had occurred to me before, and I felt like it was a good idea, but I never put aside the time—nor did I have the energy—to execute it. It reminds me of my kids' baby books. When my first was born, I was eager to fill out his baby book. I got three quarters of the way through before number two came along 15 months later. In an effort to treat all of the kids equally, I told myself I would do a baby book for child number two, as well ... soon ... but, in the meantime, would just write his information in the margins of the first baby book as a way not to forget.

The margins were as far as I got and even that was done poorly. I don't even think I got past the first two pages! There is no information documented anywhere for the rest of my kids. Ask me how long my third child was at birth and I will stare at you blankly. How old were the twins when they started crawling? Not a clue. I remember one of my best friends in college was child number three out of four children. She said there weren't many pictures of her in her parents' house and even fewer of her youngest sister. I swore I wouldn't do the same thing, yet here I was.

So, when my friend suggested I write some stories down, something clicked. Not too long ago, I had a conversation with my mom about something that happened and she replied, "Remember when this happened with one of your other kids?" The thing is, I didn't! I had no recollection of it whatsoever. Clearly my memory wasn't what I thought it was, and I realized writing things down was the only way I was going to hold on to those memories. I love the idea of journaling on paper, but am much faster at typing. So, I created a private blog to capture the highlights. I had no intention of sharing it with anyone except our family.

Around the same time, I was reading a lot of Marie Forleo's work. She created an online business course for entrepreneurs who know a lot about their trade, but not so much about running a business. That had me written all over it. I know nutrition, but not business management. I'm learning as I go.

Forleo not only runs a business school, but also gives tons of free advice weekly on how to succeed as a business owner. I highly suggest subscribing to her email list if you are looking for guidance on ways to take your business to the next level.

Her tagline at the end of all of her videos and emails is: "Keep going, because the world needs that special gift that only you can provide." After hearing that line for the umpteenth time, I started thinking about it more. What makes me different? What makes someone off the street want to come to BodyMetrix over another nutrition practice? What makes a patient request me over one of the other talented members of my staff? What is my special gift that no one else has? How can I share nutrition with a greater audience in a way that's unique, interesting, and engaging?

That's when it hit me! My stories, my life, my experiences! No one else on this planet has my unique experiences. I will admit my personal life is a little unique.

This book is a combination of stories from our crazy life supplemented by nutrition lessons that are simple and practical, yet equally powerful. You don't need another book teaching you about carbs, proteins, and fats. There are plenty of great ones out there. This book is more about execution. How do you get dinner on the table every night when you also play daily chauffeur to your kids? I can help you. How do you get your kids to eat more veggies? It's in the book! How do you eat healthy when traveling? I have tips for that too!

I also give helpful tips on how to eat. You may be thinking, "Adrianne, I may not pick all of the right foods every time, but surely I know how to put food on my fork and chew." What if I told you that *how* you eat is just as important, if not more, than *what* you choose to eat, and that by changing just a few habits, you can transform your diet? Take it from me, because doing just that radically changed the quality of my life.

Within the pages that follow, there are stories and tips about the darker side of nutrition as well. These are the thoughts that no one shares, but everyone is thinking; the stories about why we diet, the shame and guilt felt when overeating; the words we say to ourselves so easily, but would never dream of saying out loud to another person … so much of nutrition is getting out of our own heads—easier said than done, I know.

I will be raw and vulnerable. I will share my own demons and how I am working to overcome them. I will share with you the challenges of being in my profession and of being authentic with both my clients and myself. I bring these uncomfortable, often shameful, thoughts out into the open so together, we can come to a place of healing.

There are a few things you'll notice when you peruse each lesson. First, each lesson is built around the premise of *Nourishing* your soul, so that you can love yourself and be in a better state of mind when attempting to make healthy choices; *Eating* the right foods, so you can see and feel the results you so earnestly desire; and *Repeating* the practices to create healthy, long-term, yet sustainable habits.

Next, each lesson has its own theme, which is described in detail in the introductory section. This book was methodically constructed with those themes in mind, allowing you to easily follow along and take a step-by-step approach to changing your lifestyle. I recommend reading one lesson per week in order to give you enough time to implement the recommendations.

You'll also notice I'm providing two bonuses at the end of each lesson. First is a repository of action steps you are to take for the week. You only have to choose one, but there are five different styles to choose from: affirmation, action, achieve, analyze, and accountability. I do this because I am aware that not everyone gravitates toward the same style of habit formation. These five styles encompass all of the different types. If you're feeling ambitious, you're more than welcome to take a stab at doing more than one in a given week! Since some of these exercises call for reflection through journaling, I encourage you to purchase or create a dedicated healthy lifestyle journal.

These action steps are quick and easy to do and that's intentional. A lot of self-help books give you long-winded homework assignments and encourage the reader to not continue reading until the assignment is done. If you're like me, you don't have time for homework. That's why my action steps are quick and easy to achieve, but the secret behind them is building momentum. You see, I tell my patients all the time that 10 minutes of exercise is better than zero minutes of exercise. Will 10 minutes of exercise help you lose 10 pounds? No, but it will get you in the habit of being active, which builds momentum toward your desire to do a longer workout. No step is too small when you're in the process of committing yourself to a healthy lifestyle.

Finally, I'm including two "Five-Star Recipes" at the end of each lesson. So much of my practice is teaching others how to eat "more healthfully," so, I need to include the practical part: sharing recipes! I call each recipe a "Five-Star Recipe," because five out of five of my kids will eat it. I figure if all of mine will eat it—and I have some tough ones to please—you will have a good chance of getting one of your family members to eat it too.

I'm so excited to be on this journey with you. It is my hope that you can resonate with the themes of these stories and laugh at the similarities to your own life. I hope the practical tools of incorporating healthier foods into your diet will feel safe and doable even if you only make one change. Finally, it is my hope that you enjoy creating these recipes with your families while you experience crazy, lasting memories of your own to share with me too. Shall we get started?

lesson 1

Set Yourself up for Success

"You don't have to be great to start, but you have to start to be great."
—Zig Ziglar

Starting a new project is exciting. Whether it's starting a new diet, a new exercise program, or even reading a new book, there is a level of anticipation and giddiness to trying new things. We start anything new with the hope to gain knowledge and produce change. So much of our success hinges on two things: placing ourselves in a position to be successful and anticipating the roadblocks. My job as a dietitian is to help my patients create that environment and identify potential challenges. If we are able to discuss both facets in detail ahead of time, the patient is much more prepared when life throws her curveballs, and typically, she can adjust quickly and reach the goal more efficiently.

The following stories do just that. They are setting you up to be successful, both mentally and physically. As much as we want to do our best, we tend to meet the same challenges over and over again, causing frustration and suboptimal performance. Reprioritizing what is important and cultivating a foundation of solid principles sets the stage for healthy habit formation.

Getting started is exciting but it can also be scary. Taking that first step forward usually means leaving behind what feels safe and comfortable. This journey will be a collaborative effort. I am not the "expert" who shouts out orders. I am the trusted guide and friend, standing by your side the entire time. Together, we will accomplish great things and have a lot of fun along the way. So, tuck away any hesitation or worry, because we are in this together. Let's get started. Let's do this!

nourish

135, Fully Dressed

My earliest memories of a scale include watching my mom get on one every single morning. I remember thinking how beautiful she was, as she got ready for work, carefully curling her hair and putting on makeup. She frequently wore dresses and strappy heels and deliberately picked out her jewelry.

My mom dropped me off at daycare on her way to work most mornings. After she would finish getting ready (shoes and all), she had one final step left in her routine: open the door to the bathroom closet and get on the scale. Her goal was to weigh 135 pounds, fully dressed. I know this, because I heard her say it all the time. Sometimes the number on the scale made her happy and other times it made her feel sad. I learned at a very young age that the scale could make you feel many different ways.

Now, fast forward to a year or two ago. This was about the age for my two oldest boys to become aware of their body sizes. Jake and Parker are only 15 months apart and are always competing. Parker, who is younger, is actually tall for his age and most times appears bigger than Jake. Naturally, the two began to compete on both weight and height, weighing in regularly for bragging rights. Once Parker surpassed Jake in weight, the conversation changed to Jake teasing Parker about "how fat he was." Parker started asking questions about calories and nutrition labels. My husband even caught Parker weighing himself several times one day. Jim threw the scale out that day and I supported his decision, even though a small part of me felt a twinge of panic. How was I going to control my weight if I didn't see the number every morning?

There's irony in the idea that I have my own issues surrounding the scale considering my occupation and what I teach others on a daily basis. In college, I wrote a magazine article for my gym's publication about not letting the scale define our worth. I even wrote a spoof on the rules of weighing in:

1. Always weigh yourself in the morning, since later in the evening tends to be unkind.
2. Empty your bladder and/or bowels before stepping on the scale.
3. Always weigh yourself without clothes on and with dry hair (before your shower, never after).
4. Exhale so that the number on the scale says the lowest possible number.

The lengths people will go to when getting on the scale in my office are sometimes comical. I have one patient who takes off her glasses, despite the fact she is then unable to read the number on the scale. I even had a patient take off her dress pants, convinced the heavy material would skew the number.

Intellectually, we know the number does not define us, yet we sure do let it mess with our heads. See a number you don't like and it can totally ruin your mood for the day, which is a shame, because the only thing you have done up to this point is get undressed and go to the bathroom. However, see a number you do like and you feel like you're flying!

Where it gets confusing is when you see a number you like after "being bad." It messes with your head a bit and you feel like you got away with something. You start to question if you can get lucky twice and start testing the boundaries. It's even more confusing when you see a number you don't like after following all the rules. You eat "perfectly," you exercise, you drink your water, and you get enough sleep. Yet, the scale doesn't move. This particular circumstance normally leads to anger, frustration, and unfortunately for some, defeat and temptation to give up.

I often weigh my patients at the end of a session for this very reason. On a regular basis, I will have a person come into the office for his or her second appointment on cloud nine, because he or she has more energy, feels less chaotic around food, is sleeping better and notices improvements in his or her mood. All of the changes that patient made to his or her diet are positively affecting his or her life. However, if the scale doesn't reflect a change, hands fly into the air in frustration. It's time to call this off.

Hold up! You just told me how much better you're feeling, that you have more energy than you have had in months, and you're finally sleeping through the night, but it's not working?! Yes, because no matter how many times people say it's about health, it's about that stupid scale. To that, I say, it is impossible to have a good relationship with food if you are a slave to the scale. The two cannot coexist.

Not 'One Size Fits All'

There is a thing called "weight set point." We don't want to believe it exists, because every women's magazine cover tells us we can be smaller. Weight set point does exist and we need to talk about it more often.

Just like your body has a predetermined height and shoe size, your body has a weight set point. If you don't like your body's weight set point, ask yourself why. Who told you that your weight set point wasn't okay? Was it your family, your friends, your old boyfriend, your magazine subscription? It is possible to lose weight below your set point, but if it means eating 700 calories and exercising two hours per day to achieve it, then I will call you out on it. It's not healthy for you.

So, how do we make peace with ourselves and get past the emotional ties we have to the scale? We throw out the scale. When I suggest this to patients, I usually get a lot of scared looks. Even though they intrinsically know it's hurting their emotional journey with food, the scale acts as a security blanket. Giving up that security is hard! Yet, it's necessary.

If the scale is dictating your mood, your emotions, and how you talk to yourself (and others), then it needs to go away. You are more than a number. Repeat that. You are more than a number! Health is not reflected in a number. Your value isn't reflected in a number. Your worth is not reflected in a number. Scales and formulas—like those used to calculate our BMI—are tools, but they are not the end all, be all. They just produce generalized numbers, numbers that do not account for muscle. The goal is always to build muscle for weight loss, because the speed of your metabolism is based on how much muscle you have (which is why guys can look at a treadmill and lose five pounds and women have to be on it for a week to lose half an ounce).

The number on the scale also reflects fluid shifts. A muscle cell is made up of more than 70 percent water,[1] so if you start to break down muscle, you will see the scale go down due to fluid loss.

If you eat a carbohydrate one day after weeks of avoiding it and the scale goes up, it is due to fluid gain.[2] If you have a weird fetish of tracking fluid shifts all day and are okay with the results dictating your mood, then by all means, weigh yourself daily (or even multiple times a day). You will never weigh the same weight multiple times in a day.

You are more than a number.

Repeat.

You are more than a number.

eat

Hardwired

I remember the day we bought our first home. Jim and I were getting married the next month, and like many engaged couples, we had started looking for houses prior to our wedding date. We found two very nice townhomes that

4

we were considering, but at the last second our Realtor found a single home in a cute neighborhood close to Jim's work. We scheduled the first showing appointment available the next morning and it was everything I could have dreamed of in a home. I immediately fell in love with it and our offer was accepted 12 hours later.

One of the parts I was most excited about was the security system. The former owner's father owned a home security business, so I'm not exaggerating when I say this system was tricked out. I had never lived in a home with a security system, so I was dazzled by all the things it could do. One of the best features was we would never have to call 911 in the case of a fire. If the smoke alarms went off, the fire department would immediately be dispatched and our house could be saved in minutes. It even had a talking indoor/outdoor speaker system that said, "Fire! Fire! Please leave immediately," complete with sirens that would repeat until the system was shut down. I felt so safe.

Even though I love to cook, it didn't come naturally to me at first. Envisioning myself as a "good wife," I wanted to learn and try fancy cooking techniques, like braising, flash frying, and searing. The latter method requires high temperatures to create a crust on your meat to lock in the flavors for moisture, while the rest of the cooking is typically done in the oven. High temperatures tend to produce some smoke, which is unfortunate when you have a smoke detector right next to the stove.

One sunny, calm, quiet afternoon, I got home from work early and decided to sear some roast beef for dinner. Before I knew it, the smoke detector went off and lights instantly started flashing. The speaker screamed, "Fire! Fire! Please leave immediately," over and over, followed by wailing sirens at a piercing decibel level.

"Oh no! No, no, no, no, no, no! This isn't a fire, just a little smoke!"

I ran around, frantically trying to open windows to make that awful sound stop, the speaker screaming louder and louder with each second that passed. Gaining a bit of composure, I called the number for the security service to tell them to "please make this loud sound go away," which they did. Unfortunately, the fire department was already on its way.

I pleaded with the person on the other end of the line to call the fire department and tell them it was a mistake, but much to my disappointment, she repeatedly informed me (very politely I might add) that she could not do that.

I had no other option but to walk outside my front door to greet the big red truck and a few of my new neighbors that I hadn't had the luxury of meeting yet. I was mortified. The fire trucks (yes, two) came rushing down our quiet cul-de-sac only for me to tell them everything was okay, that I was just starting to learn how to cook, and that I was so sorry. They entered the house to investigate and we all politely chuckled at the incident. After they left, I called Jim at work to tell him everything, tears not withheld.

I wish I could say that was the one and only time my attempts at cooking produced an overabundance of smoke tripping off the alarm. Who in their right mind puts a smoke detector right near the stove?! I probably had the fire department at my house three or four times, with each moment mimicking the events of the first encounter.

After the third incident, there were no more polite chuckles. I can't say I blame them. There was also a smoke detector at the top of our vaulted ceiling in the family room, which was attached to the kitchen. I'm no builder, but that placement made the least sense to me. Of course, smoke will rise, but when one fireman told me to get a rag and wave it in front of the detector to clear some smoke, I told him I would need to climb a 40-foot ladder to get to that detector. That wasn't happening.

You would think all of these horribly embarrassing moments would have deterred me from cooking, but I was insistent on figuring it out. On several occasions, I called the alarm company proactively. I would tell them my name (I probably could have skipped that step since they knew me very well by then), that I was trying a new recipe which was creating some smoke, and if my detector went off to please not dispatch the fire department. Thankfully, that tactic seemed to work the best and I no longer had to meet my neighbors on the front porch.

Could you imagine those poor people inside their homes, enjoying family time, only to have it interrupted by sirens and talking security systems? As for the fire department, I heard they changed their policy to charge people for coming out unnecessarily a year after we moved out. I choose to see that as mere coincidence.

The first time the smoke detector went off in our current home, my heart immediately sank as I panicked, instinctually moving toward the phone to make the call. I let out a huge laugh and sigh of relief after realizing no one was yelling at me to the background of shrieking sirens. To this day, the smoke detector's initial beep gives me a jolt of anxiety, but it's getting better as time goes on. I'd like to think all of those experiences have made me the amazing cook I am today, or maybe it was a lesson on humbleness. Clearly, I am still in need of further education.

Rewire Your Thoughts on Cooking

When it comes to cooking, some of us are not naturally hardwired with the ability to produce tasty meals. I envy the people who just throw things together or add a little of this and a little of that. I am not one of those people. Cooking takes practice, patience, and grace. Realizing you're going to mess up along the way is part of the learning process.

I have several patients who absolutely despise cooking. Yet, it is a life skill we need to acquire for both health and survival, considering we eat several times a day. This is why I am adamant that my kids learn how to cook. I'm investing in their future health.

If you resonate with my patients that don't enjoy cooking, I invite you to change your perspective. Instead of looking at it as a chore, choose to see it as an investment. Make the experience pleasant by turning on some music, anticipating the cleanup, and inviting others to join. Crystal, a close friend of mine, doesn't like cooking, but she does like hanging out with friends, so she meal preps with her friends a few nights a month to make the process more enjoyable.

For stay-at-home moms with younger children, make dinner during naptime. Then, when the kids are melting down after the long day, you can address their needs while dinner is reheating in the oven. This tip saved me on several occasions!

In his book, *Cooked,* Michael Pollan writes that the reason Americans are overweight is because they don't cook anymore.[3] Do you agree? I have a gut feeling he's on to something and I am able to see it firsthand in my practice. My patients that eat out more than once a week struggle more with weight loss than those who eat at home. One patient in particular is in her 40s and never learned how to cook. Her options are to dine out, reheat something frozen, or piece together random prepackaged foods from the grocery store (Note: cheese and crackers is not a healthy, balanced dinner option).

Cooking at home absolutely has its benefits. First and foremost, it's cheaper, which always speaks to my frugalness. More importantly, a home-cooked meal will *almost* always be healthier. Dining out typically comes with a lot of added sugar, salt, and fat. Portions are larger, which means greater caloric consumption. When we go out to eat, we lose the opportunity to share wisdom and traditions with our family when everyone is eating a different dish. There is something powerful about creating a meal with our hands and everyone consuming the same food.

But let's pause for a moment and focus on the word "almost." Obviously, if you are choosing high-calorie preparation methods at home, this will not take you closer to your health goals. Using a deep fat fryer is not a recommended method to cook your food. Adding a stick of butter to your vegetables or baking sweet treats every night is just as unhealthy as ordering them at a restaurant. If you employ the same cooking techniques used at most restaurants, then you will still get the same results as if you visited the establishment. If you are not familiar with words like roast, broil, stir-fry, poach, or grill, buy a cookbook that teaches you all about these healthy preparation methods.

The point I want to make leading up to all of this is: don't give up! If your meal is a fail, try again tomorrow. Know that I'm cooking a meal too, right beside you in spirit (but actually in Southeastern Pennsylvania). Honestly, there's a good chance I'm even waving a dishrag in front of my smoke detector this very moment.

repeat
Herding Toddlers

In my experience, I've come across two major groups of people that struggle the most when it comes to weight loss: former athletes and people who have had success with losing weight in the past. We'll focus first on those individuals who have had prior success, because there is a valuable lesson to be learned from their thoughts and experiences. Later in the book, we'll discuss former athletes in more detail.

The reason why the successful dieter struggles so much down the road is that she remembers where she left off when things were going really well. The successful dieter remembers the discipline she had around eating the right foods and consistently working out. Health was a part of her everyday schedule and routine. The successful dieter remembers how great she felt when everything was going her way.

One day, though, something happened. It could have been a job change, a newborn baby, an injury, or a vacation. Whatever it was, it disrupted the schedule—derailed the routine. Not far behind was the struggle. There was motivation to get back into the routine, but things were different now. It was harder than the first time around. For her, it was followed by a complete and utter fall off the wagon—not a slight roll off the wagon, but a skin your knees, get medical intervention kind of fall, and over time, the wagon was soon out of her line of sight.

The story doesn't end there. A day will come when the successful dieter gets motivated again. Office challenges, the New Year, heck, even a Monday will do it, but she can't seem to find her way back to health utopia. She does all the right things the first three days. She packs her meals, throws away all the junk food, goes to the gym, keeps a journal on food intake, but then life gets in the way again and the following week, success drops off.

This week, the successful dieter may only accomplish one of the things on her list, and because most of us follow the "I'm either doing it all right or it's all wrong," approach, she gives up again. She may try it again, but she feels so overwhelmed to get it all perfect, that she gives up even faster than the last time. This only leads to more frustration, shame, and grief. Everything feels impossible.

Can you resonate with this story? I see it all the time in my office. I have to remind my patients that the reason it's harder the second, third, fourth, or 20th time around is because their expectations are such that the starting line has moved to where the finish line was before things fell apart.

The reason the successful dieter struggles is because she has an expectation that she is just going to pick up exactly where she left off, and when things don't look exactly like that, she feels like she is failing. So, she gives up.

What we often forget is life is not like *Groundhog Day*, where every single day is going to look like the one before. We will always have new challenges and new norms. What worked before may not work in the future and that is okay.

If you get so caught up in trying to make things look the way they once did, you are sure to feel overwhelmed. You can't make it look exactly the way it was before, because you are in a different time and place. You are not the same person as you were before. You may have new roles and responsibilities, which automatically makes this time different.

Choose the One Thing

I frequently present this idea to my patients, and if you have or have had toddlers, this will make perfect sense. Let's say you are going to run a race with your friends. Their names are Meal Planning, Healthy Eating, Eliminating Desserts at Night, Exercise, Stress Management, and Sleep. The plan is to all run at the same pace so you can stay together. How fun! It will be exactly like the time you ran the race last year. Your motivation and expectations are high and there is a small level of thrill as you anticipate the starting gun going off.

There's only one problem. I left out one little detail. The friends you are running with? They're toddlers. Have you ever tried to line up toddlers? It's virtually impossible. You get one toddler in position; tell him to stay in his place, turn your head for not even a second to line up the next toddler, and the first kid has already left his spot.

So, what do you do? You go back to the first toddler, tell him more sternly to stay in his position, turn your head for a second to grab the next kid, only to find the first kid has left his spot again. Herding toddlers is like herding cats. They do what they want, not what you want.

You spend so much time and energy trying to line everyone up correctly at the starting line that you have no energy left to run the actual race. After a few more failed attempts at trying to get everyone in position, it's just easier to give up.

This is what it's like when you try to get everything perfect with your diet. You will put so much time and energy into trying to line everything up perfectly to start, that you won't have any energy left to actually live the healthy lifestyle with any form of consistency. If you're spending more time trying to get everything lined up than actually putting in the work, then we need to find a new way. Lucky for you, I have the answer.

Turning Toddlers Into Ducklings

Grab the hand of one toddler. I don't care if you grab the toddler that's standing the closest to you or the one that's easiest to catch, just grab a hand and cross the start line.

If sleep is the easiest thing for you to manage right now, start there. If eating more fruit is the step that seems the most realistic to you, start there. Start somewhere and gain momentum. Start moving forward and gaining confidence. The bottom line is to just get started. Don't wait until you get it perfect.

If you're waiting for all of your toddlers to line up on their own, you're going to be waiting a really long time. What I found in my experience with kids is that if you start moving forward with one toddler, the other kids will follow.

Imagine a mama duck and her row of ducklings behind her. The mama duck starts walking and before you know it, the rest of the ducklings fall in line as if to say, "I wonder where they are going? I want to go too!"

I can still vividly recall the times we raised ducklings on our farm. It's so much fun to get them to follow you! They don't care where they are going; they just want to come along for the adventure.

It's the same with toddlers and the same with your health goals. If all of a sudden you start sleeping longer, you may find you have more energy to expend in the day. You may find you actually want to go to the gym after work, because you have the energy to do it. When you start going to the gym, you may find that you start making healthier dietary choices, because you notice you have less cramps on the treadmill after you eat a packed lunch versus when you go to McDonald's.

Instead of trying to do all of it from the beginning, you let the momentum of one change lead the way for all other positive change. Moving forward is the quickest way to change. I challenge you to ditch the "get it perfect from the beginning" mentality and just start somewhere. Don't worry about how your new normal compares with your previous attempts. Don't look behind. Just move forward!

choose your plan

Affirmation

Repeat this statement every day this week:

"My worth is not tied to the number on the scale."

Action

Do not weigh yourself this week. Hide the scale. Better yet, throw it away!

Achieve

Prepare six meals this week—breakfast, lunch or dinner.

Incorporate recipes from this book or choose from your personal cookbooks or Pinterest page. Bonus points if you turn on some music or enlist a family member for help.

Analyze

Answer the below question in your dedicated healthy lifestyle journal:

Which one of your health goals seems the easiest to attempt and attain right now?

Choose that goal today, write it down, and act on it the rest of the week.

Accountability

Answer the below questions in your dedicated healthy lifestyle journal:

What change did you attempt to make this week?

Were you happy with the results?

What challenges did you encounter?

How would you do things differently next time?

5-star recipes
Make-Ahead Omelets

Whenever I meet with a patient for the first time, we typically start by coming up with some healthy breakfast options. I'm a fan of getting breakfast in order since it sets the tone for the rest of your meals. Chopping veggies daily for breakfast can be daunting, so I recommend prepping enough to last the week. Cracked eggs should only stay in your fridge for 48 hours, so if you decide to make this recipe for the week, wait to add the eggs until the day you are cooking them.

Makes 2 servings

Ingredients

Nonstick cooking spray

4 eggs

¼ cup shredded cheese of your choice (I personally like cheddar, goat or feta)

½ cup finely chopped veggies (ex. onions, peppers, tomatoes, spinach, broccoli)

Salt and pepper to taste

1 TBS freshly chopped basil

Directions

1. Grease two 16 oz. Mason jars with cooking spray.
2. Crack two eggs into each jar. Divide cheese and veggies between the two jars and season with salt and pepper.
3. Place lids on jars and shake vigorously until eggs are scrambled and ingredients are combined.
4. Remove lids and microwave on high for 2 minutes, checking every 30 seconds after the first minute. Garnish with basil and serve.
5. If you prefer not to microwave your eggs, simply pour contents into a sauté pan and cook over medium heat on the stove until eggs are set.

Easy Pork Tenderloin

Searing meat has never been my strength in the kitchen, so broiling has become my favorite quick-cooking method. This recipe tastes amazing and frees up my appliances for other dishes when cooking for guests.

Makes 8 servings

Ingredients

    1 large or 2 small pork tenderloins
    Nonstick cooking spray
    4 TBS Dijon mustard
    3 TBS avocado oil
    1½ tsp celery salt

Directions

1. Slice the pork tenderloin on a diagonal, ¼ to ½ inch thick, to allow for the greatest surface area to be exposed. Grease a broiler pan with cooking spray and arrange the pork slices on top.

2. In a small bowl, mix the mustard, avocado oil, and celery salt. Use the back of a spoon to coat mustard mixture on top of the pork slices.

3. Broil on high for 7 to 8 minutes, flip, and broil until cooked through, approximately 6 to 7 more minutes.

lesson 2

The Practice of Patience

"It's not about having enough time, it's about making enough time."[1]
—Rachael Bermingham

Patience is not one of my defining attributes. In fact, it's probably one of my biggest challenges. I like movement and making decisions. Too often, I rush to make a decision so I can move forward to the next idea, that I frequently make the wrong decision.

Building from our foundation in the first section, we now move into why it is so important to create a healthy mindset from the start. This will be the well from which eventual expectations and actions flow. Momentum is a good thing, because it keeps us moving forward and motivation levels high. However, if we are constantly in a rush, we usually miss out on the life lessons.

This next section speaks to the virtue of patience. It teaches us lessons on staying present in the moment—both in mind and body—and creating a culture that speaks truth from the beginning. It reminds us that in order to be successful, we need to abstain from rushing through general life practices and appreciate where we are in the moment. It teaches us how to enjoy our personal journeys as well as the destination.

The stories in this next section highlight so many of my "parenting wins" (sarcastic tone), but illustrate this principle of slowing down beautifully. Life will keep moving, passing us by, unless we are adamant about grabbing the moments and holding on to them. We are tasked with this intentional decision every day. The culture you decide to create for both you and your family will ultimately determine your success.

nourish

There's Always One in the Bunch

For those of you who are teachers, Sunday school leaders, mothers of multiple kids, or caregivers in other capacities, you'll know what I'm talking about here. There's always that one kid who seems to find trouble (or trouble finds him). In our house that kid's name is Ben, my third boy and literal middle child.

My first two boys are 15 months apart and my last two kids are twins. Ben is three years younger than my second child and almost two years older than the twins. He's smack dab in the middle.

Ben is awesome. He loves life and pushes himself to new adventures. He's always ready to try new things and has an infectious smile. He's a little wild at times—a risk taker—but super smart and sweet. I can see it in his eyes when he feels lost in the shuffle and needs attention, which can happen often in large families.

Ben's also the kid who always gets hurt. He fell down the stairs when he was 12 months old, requiring a call to 911 when he lost consciousness. That might have been one of my top scary moments to date.

When he was 18 months old, he fell in the garden and just so happened to catch a rusty wire poking out from a fence in the corner of his eye. He stood there, blood gushing from his eye, as I charged at him with super speed and scooped him up. I ran, as fast as a five-month pregnant (with twins) woman could, back to the house. As luck would have it, we had a new babysitter starting that day. She pulled into the driveway as I was loading up the older kids in car seats to go to the doctor. I quickly shouted at her to get into the car and then politely made introductions.

"Hi Megan, my name is Adrianne, it's nice to meet you," I calmly stated. "The boy on the left is Jake, the one on the right is Parker, and the toddler with the bloody eye in the middle is Ben. Kids, say 'hi' to Megan."

Ben also has had his fair share of burns. There was the time he touched the lawn mower's engine, and the time his older brother spilled boiling water on his wrist, trying to make hot chocolate.

While we vacationed in Tennessee, he jumped off the top stair at the rental and twisted his ankle. We had plans to hike up to Clingman's Dome, which is the highest point in Tennessee, and Jim and I had the pleasure of taking turns carrying him up the mountain (in fact, we were dutiful in carrying him on all of our hikes that week). Even though it was only a half-mile hike to the peak, the gradient was 13 percent!

"Mom, do you know you're carrying 80 pounds right now?" he said to me during that grueling trial.

"Yes, Ben, climbing up a hill this steep wouldn't be nearly as entertaining or difficult without an 80-pound beast on my back," I gently teased. "Thank you for allowing me to experience this adventure with you!"

Don't Let Food Consume You

What part of your life needs adventure? What new experience or goal is in the back of your mind just waiting for you to explore?

The thing with food and weight loss is it can be an all-consuming force, holding us back from living the adventure we were created to experience. Filling out food journals has its place when we are trying to bring awareness to our eating habits and patterns, but it is only a tool. A behavioral therapist at an obesity conference I once attended, who was one of the speakers, made sure to hit home the point, "Tell your patients they need to get a life. This cannot and should not be the only thing they focus on."

I have to admit, I have fallen victim to this in my own journey. I get all excited creating charts, workout calendars, and food logs. I fill them out religiously, only to get overwhelmed and consumed with them. I know I cross the line when I start to get anxious at the thought of not having them filled out completely.

I once made a goal to run 18 miles a week. My schedule only allowed me three days per week to run, so missing a day meant running a lot of miles over the course of the remaining two days. One week, I was down 12 miles with only a day left. I started getting extremely agitated and anxious thinking about having to run that distance. Deep down, I knew it was ridiculous to have such intense feelings and totally okay to miss the goal one week. The more agitated I became, the more it became clear that this was starting to consume my life and become unhealthy. I needed to get a life.

How are you doing in this category? Do you frequently get hyperfocused and so preoccupied with what you're eating that it interferes with you living your best life? Do you spend so much time on food logs and workout spreadsheets that normal, everyday tasks, like unloading the dishwasher or folding towels aren't getting done? Are you missing out on social time with friends and family because you can't miss a workout?

Where do you need to take a step back and recalibrate? I tell my patients all the time that I, too, am a work in progress and am still trying to figure it all out. However, I have learned over the years that being "healthy" encompasses both physical and mental health.

It doesn't matter if you're a size two. If you're battling a war inside your head 24/7, that is not a mark of good health. That is prison. Analyze your current goals to make sure they are realistic and attainable. There's nothing wrong with pushing yourself to achieve new things—that is admirable and exciting—just make sure you don't take it too far and miss the adventure for which you were created.

If you're not sure, solicit advice from a trusted friend or mentor who understands your goals, but can look at the situation from a neutral position. When asking for advice, remind yourself to entertain the comments with an open mind instead of becoming defensive. Remember, you asked that particular friend because you trust his or her advice. Finding the balance between working toward health goals and maintaining mental sanity will look different to each person. It may take some trial and error. But with time, it will open the door to a healthy balance of long-term success and adventure.

eat

The Black Box that Melts Chocolate

Ben was four when he told me about the great day he had at preschool. He said his teacher, Miss Angie, put chocolate into this black box, pushed some buttons, and after it beeped a few times, she took it out and the chocolate was melted. He was mesmerized. You may be confused, because the year was not 1960. It was 2013. He was referring to a microwave, of course, but since we don't own one of those, he didn't know what to call that magical black box.

We used to own a microwave, before 2005, when I was pregnant with our first son, Jake. Jim heard somewhere that women shouldn't stand in front of the microwave if they were expecting, and in a very Jim way, extrapolated that information to mean if you shouldn't stand in front of a microwave pregnant, then no one should ever stand in front of a microwave. He made me promise not to reheat food in it and I reluctantly agreed.

One afternoon I needed to heat up some baby food for Jake. I knew Jim didn't want me to use the microwave to heat up the food, but heating up water in a mug to create a makeshift double broiler most certainly did not go against his wishes (or so I thought). So, this became my daily routine at meals. I didn't think much of it until the day Jim surprised me and came home for lunch.

When he saw the mug spinning around in the microwave he asked if I had been using it the whole time. I told him the truth: I was only heating up the water to heat up food, and as soon as I pushed start, I would run out of the room (maybe that last part wasn't true but the details are getting fuzzy 13 years later). This apparently didn't amuse him. He unplugged the box and threw it outside. Literally tossed it. I made him go pick it back up, because I really didn't want to be the neighbors with the microwave on the front lawn. That was the day the microwave left the premises—never to return.

When I tell people I don't own a microwave, I get some pretty confusing stares. When my friend Kristi came to my house for the first time, she told me we could not be friends because of this oddity.

It's really not so bad once you get used to it, though. We're able to heat up most foods either in the toaster oven or on the stovetop. It takes a few extra minutes, but I will say the quality of the food is much better and I no longer have red tomato sauce staining my Tupperware.

Slowing time down isn't a bad thing either. I feel like the people of my community thrive on rushing from one activity to the next, and I'm pretty sure my town looks just like yours. It's almost a badge of honor to rush around. You have to be very intentional not to get caught up in the rat race.

Rushing around has its drawbacks. The microwave was designed to save us time, but instead of using that time wisely, we're just filling that space with more things to do.

Conventional cooking has a way of slowing you down. Rush while chopping vegetables and you may find yourself in the ER with one less digit. Crank up the oven to 450° and your chicken will come out dry.

To cook well, you need to develop the art of patience. One of my favorite authors, Michael Pollan, wrote in his book, *Cooked*, "Great cooking is all about the three 'p's: patience, presence, and practice."[2] Cooking forces you to be in the moment. Society teaches us to be anywhere but. I remember when I first started interviewing for jobs, I told my prospective employers that my strength was in multitasking. Most recently, when I try to multitask in the kitchen, I find I'm not successful and end up rereading the directions three and four times to get it right.

I wish I were one of those kitchen sink cooks. You know, the kind of cook who just throws random ingredients in random amounts into a pot and the outcome is amazing; the type who never follows a recipe and just uses her taste buds to guide her journey. I'm the type who follows the recipe verbatim. Shortly after I got married, I called my mom for her pork chop sauce recipe.

19

"I don't know Adrianne," she murmured. "I just mix ketchup, mustard, and brown sugar together."

"But, how much of each ingredient? What if I put in too much of one or not enough of the other and it turns out inedible? I need the exact measurements! I need the directions!"

I quickly learned none of this mattered being married to Jim, because he puts ketchup on everything. **Everything!** I used to get so upset when I would spend hours perfecting a sauce and he would pour ketchup all over the dish without even trying it first. I'm happy to report that 15 years later, more times than not, he tries everything I make first *before* adding the ketchup. That's love, right there.

Every good, healthy recipe starts with chopping a plant in some form, whether it's onions, greens, or fresh fruit. Embrace the slower speed, stay in the moment, and know that you are treating your body kindly on many levels when you choose to cook. Your body will thrive from the abundance of vitamins and minerals, and your mind will flourish from the break of the normal rush.

Take a break from the magicical black box and try a new recipe from scratch this weekend. Enjoy the solitude and rhythmic chopping or enlist family members and create a memory. Either way, you can't lose.

repeat

'I Can't Wait to Tell Everyone What Mom Did'

My father's philosophy is to always arrive everywhere early. He has the mind-set that "on time" is considered late, so it's important to show up at least 10 minutes early. As a teenager, I would beg him to leave the house later so we wouldn't be the first people to arrive on the scene.

In my early adult years (read that as "before kids"), I kept up the tradition and maintained the early arrival legacy he passed on. That is until I met Jim and had kids. I wouldn't say Jim is late, but he's definitely not early. The kids threw a whole new wrench into our system. Jim says it's perfectly acceptable to be five minutes late per kid.

I tried to adopt the 25-minute late rule in my own life, but it just created too much anxiety. In fact, our biggest fights to this day are on Sunday mornings trying to get to church on time. We are that family having an all-out screaming match to get everyone in the car, and then five minutes later, wearing big smiles as we greet our friends walking from the parking lot to the building.

I'm a fairly organized person. In fact, I pride myself on having it together most of the time. I get completely thrown off when I think I have it together and end up forgetting something. Managing everyone's schedule is tricky, but a challenge I enjoy conquering. I only use paper calendars and write reminders one and two weeks in advance of upcoming appointments so I can mentally prepare for what is ahead. I realize my system works for me and is not for everyone.

You may be able to imagine my complete and utter confusion when I showed up to my children's elementary school one morning and there was only one car in the parking lot. This was absolutely one of those times I thought I had it together and clearly did not.

Typically Jim left for work everyday at 8:30 a.m. On this particular morning, Jim left for work a lot earlier than usual, so when I woke up to a clock that read 7:45 and didn't see his car in the driveway, I panicked. For whatever reason, I chose to focus on the numbers reflecting the minutes and neglected to look at the number representing the hour. School starts at 9:00. My head is telling me it's 8:45. We missed the bus!

Frantically, I woke up Jake and Parker. Jake was in kindergarten, Parker was in preschool, and Ben was only two. The girls were only a few months old, sleeping in their cribs. I started contemplating what to do with the rest of the kids. Should I leave the four youngest at home and run Jake to school, which was only a mile and a half away? Was Parker, at four years old, mature enough to take care of three younger siblings for the few minutes it would take me to run to the school and back? I thought about this for all of about two seconds and quickly realized that was not a good option.

While Jake was still sleeping, I managed to dress him and carry the other kids to the car. I had just enough time to get Jake to school before the minute hand reached the 12. Speeding down the road, I peered into the rearview mirror just long enough to see very sleepy, dazed children.

When I pulled into the empty lot, I thought, "Did I miss an in-service day on the calendar? Was there a delay I didn't read about?" With no time to figure it out, I screamed at the boys to get out of the car as fast as possible. I should add that Ben, Parker, and I were not appropriately dressed to be out in public.

We got to the doors of the building only to find them locked. I convinced myself that it made sense, as they were probably locked for safety reasons. I started knocking like a lunatic.

The principal greeted me at the door but looked very confused. I took it as her being perplexed by our tardiness and my impeccable attendance record. I immediately started apologizing, telling her how I overslept and that my error wouldn't happen again.

Still looking at me in confusion, she finally explained to me that school wouldn't open for another hour. We both glanced at the clock hanging on the wall, and only in that moment did I see that the clock read 8:02.

Eight! Not nine! Eight! Humiliation began to set in, as my eyes grew big, realizing the mistake I had just made. I quickly apologized (again) and ran out of the school to drive home. Thankfully, the girls slept through the whole ordeal.

As I was about to ask the boys to keep this story between the six of us, Jake blurted out, "I can't wait to tell everyone at school what mom did! We should call dad at work when we get home and tell him what happened."

I'm pretty sure I offered a few bribes, but Jake refused, looking forward to reliving the moment with everyone he encountered.

What's the Rush?

We are often rushing to get places—to appointments, to work, to whatever next big thing is on the agenda. Most of my patients are in a rush to lose weight. They procrastinate until it becomes utterly impossible to lose a specific number of pounds in a finite time frame.

I worked with a lady who told me she struggled for the past 10 years to lose one pound. One! It turns out she wasn't eating enough, so I added more calories to her day and showed her what foods to include. She came back three weeks later for her follow-up appointment and got on the scale. She lost two pounds!

"It's not working," she sighed, shoulders slumped, defeat in her eyes.

"What do you mean it's not working?" I combatted. "You haven't lost one pound in 10 years and I just got you to lose two pounds in three weeks!"

"It's not fast enough," she replied. "I should have lost more."

Hold up! Are you serious? I'm a dietitian, not a surgeon who can cut things out. It didn't matter what logic I explained to her in that moment, because she was convinced that she failed.

What are your unrealistic expectations when it comes to nutrition and health? Are you putting stress on your mind and body, trying to achieve a lofty goal in a short time frame? How's that working out for you? My guess is it's backfiring because the stress is causing you to overeat, making the initial goal further away from where you originally started.

For some, fear of an impending deadline increases motivation, but I would argue the opposite is true when it comes to weight loss. So many of my patients use food as a coping mechanism, so when stress and anxiety result from an approaching deadline, it is natural for them to engage in emotional eating.

Although procrastination is the root of the problem, how we handle the stress and anxiety that it creates is what we are going to focus on here. How can we identify if and when we are eating mindlessly? Or if we are using food to cope? One tip to try is to journal your mood whenever you eat something. Notice if you are carrying any tension in your neck or shoulders. Pay attention to your eating speed. Are you eating out of frustration or anxiety? I often recommend engaging in this exercise every time you eat. Most will argue it's only necessary when you're in a moment of stress, but I will counter that with the question, "How will you be able to recognize mindless eating in a stressed state if you can't recognize it in a relaxed, healthy state?" Meaning, if you don't practice mindfulness when things are going well, you're less likely to remember to do it when you need it the most.

In any circumstance, it's important to remember that health is not a race. It's not a competition with your neighbor. It's an individual journey that ebbs and flows with circumstance, environment, and actions. Health does not stop at the physical, but encompasses mental and emotional states, as well.

I hate to spoil the ending, but there is no final destination and no arrival point; you must learn to enjoy the journey. The moment you take the calendar and unrealistic deadlines away, you will find peace, which will carry over to your food selection. Try to keep your calendars for appointments (and maybe school start times) only.

choose your plan

Affirmation

Repeat this statement every day this week:

"Health is not a competition."

Action:

Slow down! Do not use the microwave this week. Bonus points if you make one entire meal from scratch.

Achieve

Are there any parts of your current lifestyle that show imbalance? Schedule an adventure this week, such as meeting a friend for an impromptu lunch, taking a half-day vacation, or bringing the kids to a bounce house just because (and be sure to bounce alongside them).

Analyze

Notice your mood every time you eat this week and journal it. Look for patterns or trends.

Accountability:

Answer the below questions in your dedicated healthy lifestyle journal:

What change did you attempt to make this week?

Were you happy with the results?

What challenges did you encounter?

How would you do things differently next time?

5-star recipes
Herb-Roasted Chicken

This tasty recipe takes little prep work, but does require some time in the oven (as do all amazing recipes). Cooking whole chickens is super easy and economical when feeding lots of people. I frequently make this recipe for special family get-togethers, laid back Sunday afternoons, or whenever the kids don't have a weeknight practice. This dish is also featured on the front cover.

Makes 4 servings

Ingredients

1 whole chicken (4–5 lbs.)
1 tsp dried thyme
1 tsp dried oregano
1 tsp dried sage
2 TBS olive oil
½ TBS Kosher salt
1 tsp black pepper
½ small onion, cut into wedges
½ lemon, cut into wedges
3 cloves garlic
4–5 sprigs fresh poultry herbs (preferably a combination of thyme, rosemary, and sage)
1 cup fresh Italian leaf parsley

Directions

1. Preheat oven to 450°F. If present, remove the giblets from the cavity of the chicken and place the chicken in a 9x13 dish.
2. Create an herb rub by combining dried herbs with oil, salt, and pepper in a small bowl.
3. Stuff the cavity of the chicken with the onion, lemon, garlic, poultry herbs, and parsley.
4. Using your hands, cover the chicken on all sides with the herb rub and place breast side up in the pan.
5. Cook until thermometer registers 165°F and the juices run clear, about 1 hour. If cooking a larger chicken (6- to 8-lbs.), extend cooking time to 90 minutes. Let the chicken rest 10 to 15 minutes before slicing.

Summer Zucchini Chowder

In the summer, we always look forward to picking fresh zucchini and tomatoes from our garden. This is one of my favorite soups to eat using those ingredients. Prepping the veggies will take a little bit of patience, but once you pass this step, the rest of the meal comes together in no time.

Makes 8 servings

Ingredients

2 TBS olive oil
3 cups zucchini, chopped
(about 2 medium zucchini)
1 medium onion, chopped
2 carrots, peeled and chopped
2 celery stalks, chopped
½ tsp dried thyme
⅓ cup whole wheat flour
¾ tsp salt
½ tsp pepper

3 cups low-sodium chicken broth
1 tsp lemon juice
2 cups chopped tomatoes, fresh or canned
1½ cups evaporated milk
2 cups frozen corn
2 cups cheddar cheese, shredded
¼ cup Parmesan cheese, grated
2 TBS fresh parsley, chopped
1 TBS fresh basil, chopped

Directions

1. Heat olive oil in a large pot or Dutch oven over medium heat; sauté zucchini, onion, carrot, celery, and thyme until vegetables are soft, about 6 to 8 minutes.
2. Add the flour, salt, and pepper to the softened vegetables. Whisk in the broth gradually, stirring until mixture is smooth.
3. Add the lemon juice, tomatoes, milk, and corn, and return to a boil. Reduce heat and simmer for 5 minutes.
4. Add cheese and fresh herbs just before serving. Garnish with additional fresh herbs if desired.

Source: Adapted from Simply in Season: A World Community Cookbook[3]

lesson 3

Establishing Order in Your Nest

"A goal without a plan is just a wish."
—Anonymous Proverb

Oh, how I love a good plan! Nothing excites me more than a blank page in a new, crisp notebook and carefully crafting a well-thought-out action plan to meet a specific goal. I enjoy writing to-do lists and end-of-quarter goals, and meticulously filling out editorial calendars.

There was a time in my life where I wrote out so many goals on my to-do list that I was beginning to experience a lot of anxiety. My mentality shifted from being productive to feeling suffocated. I measured my worth by the number of things I accomplished in a day instead of focusing on gratitude for the ability to work hard and impact others. The more items I crossed off my list, the more arrogant and less tolerant of others interrupting me I became (and man, kids do an excellent job at interrupting). If my perfectly created plan was not carried out to a tee, I deemed the whole plan useless.

Children, time, and maturity have a funny way of putting things back into perspective. I've realized gratitude turns expectations into appreciation. Creating a plan is still of utmost importance to our success rates, but there are ways to create balance. Just like kids, adults thrive on structure and knowing what is coming next. A plan can keep us focused and from straying too far off the path. Cultivating a well-organized plan based on your personality and preferences is key to executing your health goals, as we will see in the stories that follow.

nourish

Back Inside Your House

I live in a nice, quiet suburb of Philadelphia. It's about halfway between the city and Lancaster County, also known as Amish country. Our home borders the local high school sports fields, and although there are tons of beautiful, large houses in the area, we somehow manage to live the simple farm life. My friends used to tease me because our farmhouse and property look so out of place compared to the rest of the suburban mecca landscape.

I love my town. I love the people, the community, and how close we live to both the schools and our church. The only downside is living fairly close to a major highway. Jim was reluctant about moving here, because he didn't want to hear the traffic along the busy road everyday. I can't say I have even noticed it, because the road is a little ways off, although it is still visible from our house if you look closely through the neighboring woods. Living so close to a highway has its drawbacks. You may initially think smog and noise. Our experience has been a little more dramatic.

One vividly memorable evening, Jim was working at a chiropractic center late and wouldn't be home until 8 p.m. Jake was about 18 months old and Parker was only three months old. We had just finished dinner and were watching a show together when my friend Alyssa called me.

"Hi Adrianne," she said. "I was just driving by and wanted to let you know there are police surrounding your house. Is Jim home? I didn't see his car and wanted to make sure you're okay."

"What?!" I exclaimed. "I'm sorry, I don't understand the words you are saying right now!"

I immediately looked out my front window and sure enough, there were cops lined up in front of my house. I looked out the back window and saw police with dogs walking through our backyard.

What was going on?! I could only assume they were looking for someone dangerous. Did anyone think it would have been a good idea to check on the family living inside the house, first? Perhaps it would have been nice to inform them of what was taking place outside of their home? Just a thought.

Because the kids were so little and there was a potentially dangerous criminal on the loose, I couldn't just walk outside and casually make small talk, so I called Jim at work. He told me to go into the basement and make sure the BILCO doors were locked, so the potential perpetrator could not enter the house.

I was so confused. Why was everyone talking nonsense? I most certainly was not going downstairs into the basement! What if the killer was already hiding out down there? I realize that at that point, I had no actual information on what the person of interest did. I was just going with killer.

I told Jim he needed to come home right away. I even went so far as to make him stay on the phone with me the whole time he was driving, just in case that killer really was in our basement ready to attack. I wedged a chair under the basement doorknob to try and create a blockade.

Twenty minutes later, Jim arrived, talked to the police, and found out a man was pulled over on the highway and had drugs in his possession. When the police pulled him over, he ran through the woods toward our house, hence the reason for the dogs. Because we have another wooded area behind our house, it made sense to check there in case he was hiding out. To this day I'm not sure if they ever found him.

Crazy stuff, right? That kind of excitement is a once-in-a-lifetime experience … you would think.

A few years later, we woke up in the middle of the night to the sound of helicopters and flashing bright lights. It was summer and we had our windows open, enjoying the cool breeze as we slept, which made it easier to hear the helicopters. Jim and I looked at each other in confusion and Jim immediately went to the window to see what was going on. There were police all over our yard. Remember, we live on a farm in the middle of a suburb! What the heck was going on? Why was this happening again?

Jim went outside to find out more information only to have a policeman yell at him, "Get back inside your house, sir!" He closed the door. All we could do was wait, still in shock this was happening again. It turned out there was a drug bust up the street and the accused fled in our direction. Again, the woods made a perfect hiding place, so our house became the center of the investigation.

Finally, about two summers ago, we had just turned in for the night, windows open to enjoy the nighttime air, when we heard a car coming up our driveway, followed by the sound of flip flops approaching our house, then knocking on our door.

It was midnight. Who could be at our house this time of night? Jim peered out the window and spotted a young girl. Was she hurt? Lost? In trouble? Do we open the door? Was she by herself? Was she a decoy for a big, strong man hiding and ready to shoot us? So many questions ran through our heads.

Taking his chances, Jim answered the door. Meanwhile, I had the phone in my hand, ready to dial 911, just in case. In this particular incident, the girl appeared to be stoned and was unable to find her way home. Jim told her to call her friends and have them pick her up immediately. He closed the door and we waited. Eventually, a car turned up the driveway and picked her up. Yet another crisis averted.

Gratitude

So, what's the point in me telling you all of this? We all have wacky stories to share. Thankfully, these three instances ended without anyone getting hurt. Life has a funny way of throwing in these situations every once in a while, to make us thankful for what we have and who we have surrounding us.

Gratitude keeps our heads and hearts humble, which is something we all need from time to time. We also need to show gratitude toward our bodies. It has become the norm to body shame ourselves for areas we don't like. It has become socially acceptable and expected to compare ourselves to other people in the room. This nonsense has to stop if we want to live our best lives. We need to change our inner dialogues and look toward gratitude for what we've been given. That one part of your body you continue verbally trashing is the same body part someone else in the world is asking for in prayer.

Start a gratitude journal and see how your outlook on life changes. Include the "why" when you write down the things for which you are grateful in order to create a deeper connection to your thoughts. For example, I'm thankful for my legs, because they help me stay active with my kids. I'm also thankful for the police in our area who search my property to keep my family safe. Gratitude changes things. Try it and see if you feel the same way.

eat
Buy the Veggie Tray

If you are ever going to eat more vegetables, you have to put them on the same playing field as other snack items. Let me give you an all-too-familiar scenario:

You're starving and on the verge of passing out, because you're so malnourished (cue dramatic music). Perhaps it's after a long day at work followed by a horrible commute. Waiting for dinner is not an option, so you grab the first thing you see in the pantry (think crackers, chips, or pretzels), open the bag, and receive instantaneous satisfaction as you can literally feel your blood sugar rising to normal levels despite eating at Mach speed.

Now, let's change the scene to one where the individual chooses differently:

You're starving and on the verge of passing out, because you're so malnourished (cue dramatic music). Perhaps it's after a long day at work followed by a horrible commute. Waiting for dinner is not an option, **so you open the refrigerator**.

That broccoli looks so fresh and crisp through the glass crisper door. You grab the broccoli, take it over to the sink, wash and dry it off. Next, you grab a knife from the drawer and carefully remove the treetops from their stems and then wrap up any unused portion to place back into the fridge for someone else to eat later. **Said no one ever in the history of mankind**.

Why is the latter scenario so ridiculous? Because we are lazy creatures! When you are starving, you will not choose the tougher course. You will choose the path of least resistance. Opening up a bag of pretzels takes no time and little effort. It's instant reward. While chopping up broccoli is a great choice, it is too much work. Pretzels reign victorious.

If we want to choose broccoli, we need to put it on an equal playing field. We have to make it so ridiculously convenient, it would make no sense **not** to choose it. Enter the veggie tray.

These convenient packages provide vegetables that are washed, chopped, and placed in nice, little piles next to one another. Most people opt to only purchase these for parties, but I challenge you to think differently.

My patients often tell me they could chop the vegetables up themselves. "But do you?" I challenge. That's the million-dollar question.

All of us have the ability to cut up vegetables, but if we're not doing it, then we're really no better off.

The disclaimer here is the price of the veggie tray is a little steep, but I don't have any hesitation putting it into my cart each week, because we eat it! The kids find it convenient when packing their lunches (no more, "Mom, can you cut this for me?"), and I find it extremely helpful when packing for my day for the same reasons.

I see this scenario often as well: Patients are extremely motivated to eat healthy, so they buy every single piece of produce the grocery store offers (that's a good thing). However, because of the lack of time and the effort needed to prepare the vegetables, the produce becomes overlooked in favor of the pantry. Finding moldy produce in the fridge during clean-out day reinforces why patients don't buy produce: because no one eats it and it's a waste of money. So, patients go back to not purchasing it at the store and therefore, stop eating produce.

The best part about a veggie tray is that if any vegetable begins to look questionable (limp and lifeless), you can roast it in the oven for dinner that night! This way, there's no waste!

That terrible witching hour after work before dinner is a perfect opportunity to put out the veggie tray. I find if I set it out while I'm cooking, I'm more likely to eat more vegetables, and so too are my kids and husband.

How many times do family members walk into the kitchen while you're cooking dinner, whining, "I'm hungry..." and then they either try to snatch a sample of dinner or head to the pantry to fill up on junk (and then, big surprise, are conveniently not hungry for dinner)? Throw the veggie tray on the counter and problem solved.

In my house, I would estimate 50 percent of the time the kids walk out of the room and declare they will just wait until dinner (fine with me) and 50 percent of the time they grab a stool and start noshing. What is the worst thing that can happen? They will fill up on veggies and then not be hungry for dinner? This is still a parenting win.

Take a Dip into a Pool of Options!

The top question on everyone's mind is, "What about the dip?" To that, I say, "What about it?"

If it means you and your family eat more vegetables, go for it! This is not a battle worth fighting.

In my personal experience, kids who dip veggies are more likely to eat veggies without dip later if not provided. Why? Simply put, this is due to exposure. They are used to seeing the vegetables and aren't thrown off by the lack of dip. I tried this experiment in my own home and found similar results. Sometimes the kids will ask for dip and I'll tell them there is none (that may or may not be true). Most times, they just shrug their shoulders and eat it anyway. Another win!

We know for a fact that vegetables are low-calorie, nutrient-dense, fiber-rich powerhouses. They absolutely need to be part of our diets on a daily basis. Please do not let dinnertime be the only meal of your day that you add vegetables to the menu. God forbid you run out of time or energy to make dinner as planned and end up grabbing a pizza instead. You would go a whole day without vegetables (my heart is racing, even as I type this) and that would be a travesty. Try to include them at breakfast and lunch by adding them to your eggs, on sandwiches, or as a salad.

In order to encourage my family to eat more vegetables, I do my best to make two different options for every dinner. When you have a large family, it's pretty much a guarantee someone won't like what you've cooked, but that doesn't bother me one bit. I tell them that when they get older, they'll get to cook whatever they want; that's one of the perks of being an adult.

My kids do not have to eat both vegetables, but they are required to eat at least one. If any (or dare I say *all*?!) of them likes both options, even better! If you only make one vegetable and your child (or spouse) really despises it, then you have a battle on your hands.

The only time my kids get a free pass on the prepared vegetables is if they truly hate both. I try my hardest not to do this, but it does happen on occasion. We have a clear understanding if this occurs, they can break out the veggie tray and eat from that. Again, they are eating vegetables and I'm not prepping or cooking another option. Big picture, people: choose your battles.

The more exposure your family has to vegetables, the more they will eat them. I get comments frequently from others how my kids are such "good eaters." This was a labor of love. I did not win the lottery and bear children that just magically love their veggies. I make sure to expose them to many varieties all day long. Eating vegetables is as common an occurrence in my house as watching TV. Believe it or not, my kids' favorite place to go out to eat for lunch is a diner that sells soup and salad. Parker will only buy school lunch if it's salad day (okay, maybe I won the "good eater" lottery with him).

If you want to eat more veggies, you have to make them easily and readily available to choose. If you don't like the work involved, take the shortcut and buy the veggie tray.

repeat

Baby A

I told Jim we were pregnant with twins in a public place. At that point in our lives, Jim was working crazy hours and I was home with the kids for most of the day. I taught nutrition classes one or two nights a week, and on those nights, we would frequently meet somewhere between our two jobs to hand off the kids.

That particular night, Jake and Parker had tee-ball practice at a nearby park, so the plan was for Jim to meet me at practice and from there I would drive to work. Ben was approximately 16 months old, sitting in his stroller, and I was trying to keep him entertained while the older boys were picking dandelions from the outfield.

Earlier that day, I had an ultrasound scheduled to determine a due date for the pregnancy. Since I had had three previous pregnancies, I told Jim to save his vacation time and that I would go the ultrasound myself.

"All they're going to do is make sure they see a baby and give me a delivery date," I assured him. "No big deal. You've been to them before, so it shouldn't be any different."

When I arrived at the hospital, the nurse took one look at me and then at her paperwork. She asked me if I was sure I wasn't further along than seven weeks. I immediately thought how rude that was and tried to defend my growing belly. I told her it was my fourth pregnancy and that people tend to show earlier with each successive pregnancy as if this was her first day on the job.

Shrugging, she instructed me to lie down on the table so she could get started. We exchanged small talk and then all of a sudden, she burst into laughter. I remember thinking her behavior was odd, but at that point, I was just thankful for the break from the kids and to have an adult conversation.

She stopped moving the wand on my belly, directed her attention toward me—her eyes and smile as wide as could be—and asked, "Do you want to know why you're so big?"

Again, lady, why all the comments about my size? I told you it was my fourth pregnancy!

She continued, "There are two babies in there."

What?! Did she just say **two** babies?

She turned the screen to face me so I could see the two small, white blobs in the middle of the black screen. The expression on my face must have been priceless. I shot up in the bed and grabbed the screen to get a closer look. The thought hadn't even entered my mind as a possibility at that point. I'll admit, with the first two pregnancies I remember daydreaming at the thought of twins, but not now! I already have three kids. This would make **five!**

Looking at the tech, I frantically told her she didn't understand. It's not like this was our first and second baby, or even numbers two and three. This was **four** and **five!** The news only made her howl even louder. Next thing I know, she started calling her fellow nurses over to enjoy the news.

"Laura, you've got to get over here and check this out!" she beckoned. "These are numbers four and five!" Before I knew it, I had a small crowd surrounding me, offering congratulations.

It turns out Jim should have come with me to that ultrasound so we could have enjoyed that news together, but God has a funny way of making things work out. Jim would have been content with two kids, so giving him the news that we were pregnant with numbers four and five was going to have to be handled delicately.

I decided to tell him in a public place just in case his reaction wasn't appropriate. I convinced myself that telling him in the presence of others would guarantee his excitement and tap into his calm, rational side.

When he arrived at the ballpark, I asked him if he wanted to take a lap around the parking lot with Ben and me. With a reluctant stare, he agreed. I didn't really have a plan on how I would tell him. I figured I'd just go with the flow.

"So, I wanted to talk to you about the ultrasound," I began.

"That's right. How did it go?"

"Well, there is some news we need to talk about..."

Jim stopped, "Oh no. What did they say? Is there something wrong with the baby?"

I smiled, "No. The baby is okay. It's just that Baby A isn't as far along as we thought."

Looking confused, it was obvious to me that he was stumped.

"What did you say?" he pressed.

"Baby A isn't measuring seven weeks," I replied. "Only six weeks and four days."

The confused look remained on his face. I decided to just let the weight of my words sink in for a few moments.

Eyes widening, he started to catch on, "Did you just say 'Baby A?'"

"I did. But don't worry, because Baby B is measuring at seven weeks and one day."

I couldn't contain my excitement. I was smiling ear to ear.

His wild eyes darting across my face, he stammered, "How many more are in there? Is there a Baby C?"

I chuckled, "Don't worry, silly, of course not. There's only two!"

Looking off toward the older boys, Jim grew silent. I could tell he was thinking, so I waited him out. A few moments later, he went into planning mode, mumbling about the kids needing to share bedrooms and asking himself, "Is the minivan big enough?"

I showed him the ultrasound pictures as proof and then handed him the stroller, telling him I had to leave if I was ever going to get to work on time. I can only imagine the thoughts running through his mind that night while I was at work. It makes me giggle just thinking about it!

When Life Doesn't Go as Planned

I never planned for five kids, but I am so thankful for each and every one of them. I often teach patients about meal planning as a strategy to stay on task with their nutrition goals. Just like coming up with a plan is important, it's also important to come up with a backup plan, or as I call it, Plan B. Eating out should never be Plan B. That's Plan C. Confused? Let me explain.

Plan A is your meal plan. It's what you pre-decided to make at the beginning of the week. It has all three components of a healthy meal present: lean proteins, high-fiber starches, and lots of vegetables. Plan A is what we strive to accomplish every single evening.

Plan B is an easy meal you can prepare that takes 10 minutes or less to pull together. Some of my favorite Plan B meals are scrambled eggs with veggies and whole-wheat toast, or spaghetti and frozen meatballs with a bagged salad. Another great Plan B meal can use frozen precooked chicken breasts, instant brown rice, and a bag of frozen, mixed vegetables. Plan B is super easy and quick.

Plan C is eating out. It is the absolute last option. The problem with making dining out your Plan B is that you will most likely go out to eat often, because life is fabulous at throwing curve balls (and dining out typically isn't conducive to meeting health goals).

I personally always try to have two Plan B meals in my kitchen at all times to keep us eating at home more. It's not always the popular plan with the kids, but it keeps us on budget and eating healthier foods.

One question I get often is, "My Plan A meals already are very simple. If I can't find time to prepare them, then what?"

Plan A and B meals will look different for each family based on culinary skill level and time to prepare. There are absolutely no rules (or guilt) with what Plans A and B look like to you and your family. If Plan A is already simpler in nature, then Plan B may look like frozen or pre-prepped dinners from your grocery store (some grocery stores in my area have a section where fresh meals are already prepared; all you have to do is heat them up). Rotisserie chickens are a great option in addition to the grocery's salad bar. If you are purchasing frozen meals, aim for ones with the lowest amounts of sodium.

Do you have a Plan B? More importantly, do you even have a Plan A? Do you eat out more than once a week due to changes in your schedule? This week, try stocking your freezer and pantry with a few Plan B meals and see if you notice a difference in your health and wallet!

choose your plan

Affirmation

Repeat this statement every day this week:

"I am thankful for _____

(insert body part)

because _____ *"*

(insert reasons)

Action

Buy the veggie tray this week. Bonus points if you cook two vegetables with dinner this week.

Achieve

Stock your freezer and pantry with two Plan B meals this week. If it helps, write them down and post them on your refrigerator door as a reminder.

Analyze

Take notice of your inner dialogue when it comes to your body shape. Do your negative comments outweigh the positive ones? What is your mood like following your comments?

Write your answers in your journal.

Accountability

Answer the below questions in your dedicated healthy lifestyle journal:

What change did you attempt to make this week?

Were you happy with the results?

What challenges did you encounter?

How would you do things differently next time?

5-star recipes

DIY Pizzas

When looking for a quick Plan B meal, look no further than making your own pizzas, which is kid friendly and much healthier than ordering out.
Makes 1 serving per pizza

Ingredients

Whole-grain naan flatbread
Spaghetti sauce
Mozzarella cheese

Optional Toppings
Sautéed onions
Sautéed peppers
Sautéed mushrooms
Ham
Pineapple
Miniature pepperoni

Directions

1. Throw each member in your family a naan flatbread, Frisbee style (this is important, so don't skip this step). Make sure your kitchen floor is clean beforehand.
2. Let each family member spoon sauce onto his or her flatbread.
3. Top with cheese and additional toppings of your choice.
4. Bake at 350°F for 10 minutes or until cheese is melted.

Salad Bar with Fresh Balsamic Dressing

*Believe it or not, my kids **love** salad bar night. They enjoy selecting their own top-pings and I love that they are eating all those healthy veggies. Below are the top-pings we use, but feel free to make this salad your own by choosing a variety of dif-ferent veggies, fruits, nuts, and seeds. I purposely try to choose veggies not found on the veggie tray so we don't get bored. The dressing recipe below is my go-to salad dressing 9 times out of 10.*

Serving amounts based on your ingredients

Ingredients

For the Salad
   Boxed spinach (plastic, clamshell package found in produce aisle, normally with the salads)
   Tomatoes, sliced or diced
   Garbanzo beans, rinsed and drained
   Hard boiled eggs, sliced
   Grilled chicken, cut into bite-sized pieces
   Avocado, sliced
   Craisins or Dried Apricots
   Pumpkin Seeds
   Granny Smith Apples, diced

For the Dressing
   ¼ cup balsamic vinegar
   1 TBS Dijon mustard
   ½ tsp. salt
   ½ tsp. honey
   Dash black pepper
   1–2 cloves garlic, minced
   ½ cup olive oil

Directions

1. Place salad bar toppings in bowls, or arrange on large plate.
2. Mix together all dressing ingredients in a Mason jar, cover with lid and shake to combine well. Add to salad bar toppings when ready.

lesson 4

Preparing to Leave Your Comfort Zone

"If you fail to prepare, you are preparing to fail."
—Anonymous Proverb

We now know planning is key to success with health and nutrition. At home, there is a level of comfort, because we are in our safe environment and don't need to pretend to have it all together. Out there though, *that's* a different story.

Building on the preceding section, it's time to take our plan for success from inside our home out into the real world, where challenges abound exponentially. This is where your planning skills will shine. It's what separates the prepared from the unprepared—the successful from the challenged.

This is where most people stumble. Creating a plan, or at minimum, putting some forethought into how you will behave, is paramount to a successful execution. Choosing to spend just a few minutes each day to design a game plan will help you avoid the inconvenience of scrambling at the last minute to figure things out. This practice ultimately will bless you with the gift of time and mental sanity. Most importantly, it will free you from having to make the hard decisions in the moment.

One of the best ways I can illustrate this idea is to use the example of packing your bag for the hospital early when you are having a baby. I listened to that advice the first three times. The last time, I wasn't so lucky, and the results were disastrous. I can't wait for you to laugh at my expense, but also identify with the core principles this section illustrates.

nourish

Breakfast with the Girls

Having a girlfriend with whom you can openly experience your struggles is a gift. Finding a community of people with which you can share memories and ideas, laugh and cry, and where mutual respect holds you all equally accountable, is nothing short of a small miracle. If you have a group that allows you to be transparent and the truest version of yourself, with no strings attached to your friendship, you've hit the jackpot in this soul-satisfying experience.

Our Creator calls us into community, and when done with honesty and intention, community is one of the most amazing experiences I have ever encountered.

I grew up an hour from where I currently live. I met my husband while I was in college, but since he already had a house and job, it only made sense that I move to his town after we got married. I didn't know many people other than a few people at church and work. His friends became my friends and that was that. It wasn't until Jake was born that I understood the word "loneliness." The days were long and being a stay-at-home mom meant that I didn't get out much.

It was too hard to organize my day around feedings and naps, so I just gave up and stayed in. I'm more of a homebody to begin with, so it didn't bother me too much; but it was still lonely, especially when my husband didn't get home from work until 7:30 at night.

Jim introduced me to a new coworker's wife who had just had a baby right before Jake was born. They started going to our church and she invited me to come to a playgroup on Friday mornings that our church had just started. I decided to challenge my natural introvert and was relieved to find a place of friendship, support, and laughter.

What started out as four moms quickly grew to more than 20 over the years, and it felt so nice to be part of a group that understood the challenges of being a new mom and love you through it without judgement. Looking back, I didn't realize how much that Friday morning playgroup meant to my sanity and me. To this day, the women I met in that Friday morning playgroup are my closest friends.

For the past year, I have been meeting monthly for breakfast on Saturday mornings, at 7 a.m., with three of my closest friends. We catch up on what's going on in our lives, talk about our struggles, and laugh a lot! We're committed to both our meetings and supporting each other through every-day victories and challenges.

Recently, we have started adding small road trips to our meetings. Crammed in a small room with 10 other smelly women, our first hot yoga experience together involved doing poses only gymnasts are meant to perform. To celebrate Sara's birthday, we made crafts (you will soon come to know how I feel about that). Regardless of my personal feelings, I would make crafts everyday with Sara, because she is my friend and she enjoys doing it. Our group has been through cancer scares, job changes, parenting failures, moving, foster babies, and personal successes. Meeting with these ladies is always the highlight of my month.

Leave Your Representative at Home

During our time together, there is one rule to which we've all agreed. We have each committed to never bring representatives to a group outing.

We humans bring a representative with us everywhere we go. It's the self we think others want to see versus how we really feel inside. Leaving our representatives at home is raw transparency at its core and it's scary. However, it's real, and if we are honest, real is what we crave and need from each other.

So many of my patients bring representatives to my office. They tell me what they think I want to hear, which hurts not only potential progress, but also our relationship.

I can't be helpful in the way they need me to be, because they don't tell me the scary, vulnerable stuff. A couple years ago, I saw a patient who had seen one of my colleagues a few weeks prior. She stormed into my office, claiming the other dietitian wasn't much help to her. She went on and on about my colleague's incompetency. My colleague told the patient she was doing really well with her food selections and that there weren't many suggestions she could make for change.

I took a peek at her initial intake form and her 24-hour food recall. According to the chart, the patient told my colleague she eats egg whites and fruit for breakfast, a salad with lean protein at lunch, and more vegetables and lean proteins for dinner with a small serving of high-fiber starch. I read this aloud to the patient and she sheepishly smiled back.

"Well, maybe I exaggerated what I eat in a day."

Once she opened up and was honest about her eating habits, I could give her the proper tips and tools to better help her. I completely understand the vulnerability honesty brings, but it's the only road to true healing.

This patient isn't the only one who experiences challenges. I go through my own personal struggles when my girlfriends and I go out for dinner. Every once in a while, we will order a dessert to share, but I find this particular act challenging. Typically, each lady digs in with her spoon or fork, leading to the awkward point where there are a few bites left. My friends have no problem setting their forks down and leaving the unfinished bites on the plate. I, on the other hand, have an internal battle, all the while pretending I'm okay with it, when in actuality I'm freaking out at the possibility of the waitress clearing the table and leaving two perfectly good bites go to waste.

Completely irrational, I know, but there you have it—no representatives here. When I shared this completely vulnerable story with my friend, Crystal, I was surprised when she didn't laugh or make fun of my irrational behavior. Instead, she looked at me with kindness and sincerity, and said, "How can we help you not feel this way anymore?"

Eventually, she came up with the idea of asking for four plates when we share a dessert and splitting the portions right away. Since I don't have any desire to eat unfinished food off other people's plates, this seemed like the perfect solution, and it was! I'm so glad I left the representative at home and could come to a place of resolution.

Imagine what your life would be like if you didn't bring your representative along with you. What areas of your life could find healing or provide healing to others? We are absolutely designed to live in community with one another. In the words of my pastor, "What if needing each other wasn't a sign of weakness, but a sign of awareness?"

eat

Dishonest Traveling

By now, you may have picked up on how much I love Jesus, but we all have to tell a lie from time to time. One of those times is when you're traveling with a large family. Technically, only four people should occupy a hotel room at a time, but that would mean we would have to buy two rooms. There isn't a place in the budget for that.

A few years ago, we traveled overnight to my oldest son's lacrosse tournament in New Jersey. The inn had strict rules about the number of people staying in a room, so we strategically planned our entrances and exits from the room throughout the day. The hotel had a pool, so we even went as far to pretend we were two different families and not associate with each other to conjure up the image that we were not together.

Don't worry though. Jesus had his chuckle at our expense when we came up with the idea of sleeping three to a bed. Jim and I each took two kids and one child volunteered to sleep on the floor. Looking back, I wish I had volunteered for that floor spot over sleeping in between two restless kids for eight hours. Let's just say no adult slept well that night.

In general, travel is expensive between fuel and lodging, but when you add the expense of dining out, it can tip the scales (no pun intended).

We recently bit the bullet and budgeted a trip to Great Wolf Lodge, an indoor water park in the Poconos. We spent the day enjoying the attractions and then went to dinner off site (again to save money). Afterward, we headed to the grocery store to buy food for breakfast and decided to take the kids out for some ice cream. We passed a Friendly's on the way to the grocery store and planned to get dessert on the way back, despite Jim and I not visiting the establishment in more than 20 years.

The waitress sat our family and we all began to look at the menu. Not only were the sundaes expensive since we were multiplying everything by seven, but it was hard to convince the kids to get single scoops of ice cream after looking at the sundae menu.

At this point, the kids were fighting over crayons and Jim was complaining about spending $60 on dessert. So, I did what any good mother would do. I got up and walked out of the restaurant. Never mind the fact that my kids had drawn all over their coloring pages and the waitress was on her way back to our table with seven waters. I was done. Thirty seconds later, I saw Jim and the kids walk out to the car. We ended up back at the grocery store to buy a small container of ice cream and spoons. Not our finest moment, I'll admit, but it was the best decision for us, both financially and calorically.

Ten Tips for Traveling Healthy

A good deal of my time at my practice is spent discussing how to travel healthy. Let's face it, more and more people are traveling for work and pleasure these days, so if it is going to be a big part of our lives, it makes sense to figure out how to do it in the healthiest way possible. Here are my top 10 tips for healthy, low-budget traveling:

1. **Find a grocery store first**—Google is great for this. Whenever possible, choose hotels within walking distance from grocery stores, especially when you are not planning on renting a car. Not only will it be convenient to shop, but you will also get in some extra exercise

45

between walking and carrying the groceries.

2. **Ensure a fridge**—Choose hotels with a refrigerator. Refrigerators are great for storing healthy perishables and last night's leftovers. Plus, the freezer section can hold ice packs for packing healthy foods the next day.

3. **Convenience is key**—Load up on pre-washed, chopped fruits and veggies from the produce section, individual-serving-sized yogurts and cottage cheese, hardboiled eggs, and 100-calorie packs of nuts.

4. **Breakfast in bed**—Always eat breakfast in your hotel room. Breakfast foods can be expensive and high calorie when dining out and can usually be easily prepared inside your room. Choose whole-grain cereals with low-fat milk, whole-grain miniature bagels with natural peanut butter, or yogurt parfaits with fresh fruit and granola. Use the coffee maker to heat up water for individual oatmeal cups. Pack your NutriBullet or blender to make smoothies.

5. **Go off site**—Look for restaurants outside of the establishment. Depending on where you are staying, this is helpful for your wallet and your waistline. If you're traveling with a group of people, opt to order and eat family style versus each individual getting his or her own meal, since portion sizes are generally large. In our family, we always order an appetizer, one or two dinner salads, a main meal, a sandwich of some sort (usually a burger and French fries), and then split it all once it comes to the table. We all get a taste of everything, but not a high-calorie meal that leaves us feeling sluggish.

6. **Only one luxury**—When dining out, choose one, not all three: drinks, appetizers, or desserts.

7. **Minimize stops**—When traveling by car, pack a cooler with meals instead of stopping on the way. Did you ever drive on a highway and notice there is a McDonald's at every … single … exit? I have yet to see a Saladworks advertised on a billboard. No wonder we have an obesity crisis in our country! McDonald's has done an excellent job surrounding us with quick, easy, junk food. Whenever our family travels any considerable distance, we pack a cooler with meals and snacks to last us until we arrive at the destination. I always pack a gallon-size bag of fruit and veggies (each gallon bag has three to four sandwich bags filled with different varieties of produce), as well as the main meal. I typically pack a loaf of whole grain bread, mustard, sliced fresh turkey breast, and single-serve yogurt packs. I usually line up the kids on the sidewalk with their food while Jim is getting gas just to save time.

8. **Maximize steps**—Use rest stops as activity stops instead of eating opportunities. Get out, stretch your legs, or maybe walk around the building a few times. Get back in your car and move on toward your destination. Do not let the vending machines or fluorescent lights in the food court suck you in.

9. **Make an exception**—Nutrition bars can be your friend. I'm not a huge fan of consuming them on a daily basis, because I feel they take away from opportunities to eat real, live foods, and are often loaded with sugar, making them glorified candy bars. However, since there is no such thing as a bad food, there is a time and place for bars in our diets. Traveling is one of those set times. When you need a non-perishable snack or meal idea, bars can become your go-to choice. Whether in your car or hiking on a mountain, most bars offer a decent amount of energy to get you through until your next meal.

10. **Don't forget to hydrate!**—I cannot stress water enough! Hydration during travel is so important. Most people dehydrate themselves so they don't have to make frequent stops along the way. Always fill a water bottle (or two) for your travels and keep a gallon water jug and ice in your cooler for an inexpensive refill.

So, there you have it. You are now prepared and set up to succeed when it comes to eating well on the road. As for getting a good night's sleep when your party exceeds the number of beds available, you're on your own.

repeat
Pack Your Bag

It was a Wednesday morning and I was 30 weeks pregnant with the twins. I was at my Bible study that day and the ladies in the group told me I didn't look so good. If nothing else they had the honesty part of friendship down, because my looks matched the way I was feeling.

I had a doctor's appointment scheduled at noon that day and was supposed to head into work for a few hours after. During my appointment, my doctor informed me I had already started dilating and she urged me to go straight to the hospital. My favorite obstetrician in the practice just happened to be at the hospital that day and very calmly told me the babies couldn't get the care they needed at my small community hospital. We would need to leave immediately by ambulance to a level one NICU approximately 25 minutes away.

This must be a mistake, I thought—30 weeks was too early to deliver—I was only having stabbing back pain every two to three minutes, not constantly. Surely, this was nothing to be concerned about and we were all being over-dramatic here, right? I didn't have back labor with the boys, so this was all new to me.

They gave me some magnesium to buy some time. My doctor proceeded to tell me that there was a possibility I could deliver in the ambulance.

Hold up! What?!

A few minutes later, three men walked into the room and introduced themselves as the crew that would be taking me to the other hospital. They all looked scared out of their minds! Let me tell you, there is nothing less comforting than going into labor 10 weeks early, with twins, and having to put your babies' lives in the hands of three men who looked like they never saw a pregnant person before.

Thankfully, the nurse assigned to my room agreed to ride along in the back of the ambulance to help out if needed. The nurse put her hand on my belly while we were riding down the highway. One of the men in the ambulance asked what she was doing, to which she replied, "Timing her contractions." I asked if he ever delivered twins before, to which he replied that he had never delivered any babies before. The nurse and I both prayed.

Fortunately, I made it to the hospital and the magnesium stopped my contractions. It only bought us about 36 hours, but we were hopeful it would afford us enough time to get some steroids into my system to help with lung maturity.

I was so out of it from the meds, but felt better once Jim met me at the hospital with an overnight bag and a stack of baby names I printed off the internet three months prior. We were 10 weeks out and still hadn't confirmed name options. We didn't know the sex of the twins, so we had to come up with eight names (first and middle). Since we had three boys already, the girl names came really easy to us. Boy names, not so much. All I have to say is—thank you, Jesus—for giving us two girls, because our boys would be in therapy for the names we came up with that night. I was all drugged up and Jim was sleep deprived, which pretty much meant I was the most coherent.

We delivered two beautiful girls about 40 hours later. The whole entire operating room cheered, because they knew we wanted to be surprised with the sex and they knew we already had the boys. Of course, with the prematurity, they whisked the girls off right away to the NICU and Jim followed. I was sent to the post-op recovery room. Jim checked in on me an hour or so later. He looked at me and oh so lovingly said, "What do you think about this?"

I was confused. "What do I think about what?"

"Two girls."

"I think it's wonderful. It's amazing! Aren't you so excited?"

"Eh..."

"What?! Eh?"

"I mean one girl would have been okay, but two? I'm not sure."

"It's not like we can send one back and trade her in for a boy."

Who are you and are we really having this conversation? The only thing that saved him in that moment was that I was literally numb from the chest down. I love his honesty, but his inner thoughts really need to be challenged from time to time.

It had been more than three days since my body had experienced a shower and my long hair had felt the teeth of a comb. Since Jim was home with the boys, I was alone at the hospital. I inspected the overnight bag Jim brought me, checking to see if everything I needed was there.

Slippers, check. Underwear, nope. Maternity pants and shirts, not one piece. Don't lose hope, my friends. What Jim did pack was a half t-shirt I wore in college from the university I attended and regular sweatpants. Not maternity sweatpants that would have a forgiving waistline, but fitted sweatpants that people wear before they are old enough to have children.

I started laughing at his sense of humor, because clearly this was a joke ... except it was not. This was all he packed me. To top it all off, there was no comb or brush. I just spent the past three days on bed rest and my hair was a nasty, tangled mess.

Thankfully, my friend bought me one of those small, black combs from the gift shop and it took me more than an hour to comb out my matted hair. I could not leave my room wearing the controversial clothes, so I rummaged through the cabinets and found a robe to put on over top of my suggestive outfit. When I went over to the NICU to visit the girls, the nurses had a good ole belly laugh at my unfortunate outfit. This is why every *What to Expect When You're Expecting* book tells you to pack your bags early. This is the very reason, ladies. Do not let this happen to you.

Fail to Plan, Plan to Fail

What can we possibly learn about nutrition from this experience? Fail to plan, plan to fail, and failure was written all over my outfit. When it comes to nutrition, meal planning is one of the most important things you can do for yourself and your sanity. There is nothing worse than trying to figure out what to cook at 5 p.m. when everyone is hungry and tired. It's like walking into an episode of *Chopped*, but worse, because in your reality, you have people whining and hanging onto your legs, and now you have to try to create a meal that's both nutritious and edible.

The time it takes to meal plan at the beginning of the week does not even compare to the time and mental sanity it will save you at 5 p.m. throughout the week. Instead of staring blankly into your refrigerator and pantry, you will already know what you are preparing and can get right to work. For whatever reason, planning a meal and cooking it at the same time is hard work. That's why I emphasize meal planning. With the hard work of creativity behind you, your only goal at 5 p.m. is execution.

I also suggest creating your grocery list while meal planning so you can be sure all the ingredients are ready and available when it's time to cook. Meal planning saves you money as you are only buying ingredients you need versus what looks good on an end cap.

Perhaps one of the best reasons to meal plan is that your family will complain less about the meals. I didn't say stop complaining; just complain less. The secret to this is to display the meal plan either on a chalkboard or on your refrigerator. Posting the plan for all to see gives everyone time to mentally prepare for what is coming versus having random food placed in front of them every night.

I absolutely encourage you to meal plan with your entire family since everyone will be eating the same foods. This not only teaches them the art of meal planning, but allows for each member to voice his or her preferences. In my household, when I ask family members for ideas, I usually hear crickets or am met with the response "I don't care" or "Whatever you think." I have found that threatening lentil soup for every meal usually gets their creative juices flowing, and in no time, they are able to provide productive suggestions.

Recently, Parker brought me an Asian recipe he wanted me to prepare and so we sat down together to see how we could integrate the recipe into the weekly meal plan. It was a great opportunity to dialogue with him about what I look for in a recipe when choosing to make it for our family.

The recipe he selected looked amazing but had some unfamiliar ingredients that were only needed in small amounts. We discussed how cost is a factor that I also consider when making meals and we researched less expensive ingredient substitutions for a more practical alternative.

Finally, meal planning means that you will have a better chance at executing a nutritious, balanced plate. My patients looking for weight loss and overall healthier eating are successful when they meal plan, because they have put in the forethought compared to those patients who struggle, because they are trying to figure it out as they go. My meal planners have vegetables on their plates, because they planned for them to be there. Instead of struggling to create a cohesive meal, the three components of a balanced plate (protein, starch, vegetable) are present, because they purchased and prepared them.

My meal planners are never caught off guard, leaving mealtime up to chance. They know which meals will be eaten at home and which ones will be eaten on the run. They pack healthy snacks with them in their cars and their purses. Remember, fail to plan, plan to fail. I have yet to meet a person who was successful just winging it.

Meal planning is always the common divider between those who succeed and those who struggle. Creating a meal plan will help you too, and I've included the one I use frequently in Appendix A. When I'm feeling lazy, I use the back of one of my kids' returned homework sheets, write "S, M, T, W, Th, F, Sa" on it, and start filling in the blanks. Remember, it doesn't have to be fancy or complicated. It's a simple task that takes roughly 20 minutes and has a profound impact on our well-being. I invite you to try it and see the difference it makes in both your week and your overall health.

choose your plan

Affirmation

Repeat this statement every day this week:

"I choose to show up as myself, not my representative."

Action

Create a meal plan for the following week. Either use pen and paper or an app, such as Mealime or FoodPlanner, if you prefer to keep everything digital.

Achieve

Begin to leave your representative at home and show up as yourself. This can look like opening up to a sibling or trusted friend about something with which you are struggling, talking about a goal you want to accomplish or a decision you're trying to make.

Analyze

Which traveling tip(s) would you like to try the next time you are on a road trip? Decide which one fits best for you, write it down in your journal, and make sure you consciously make an effort to use it on your next excursion.

Accountability

Answer the below questions in your dedicated healthy lifestyle journal:

What change did you attempt to make this week?

Were you happy with the results?

What challenges did you encounter?

How would you do things differently next time?

5-star recipes

Fruit and Oat Granola Bars

These granola bars are perfect for traveling and have just the right balance of oats and sweetness.

Makes 12 servings

Ingredients

Nonstick cooking spray
1 cup quick-cooking or old-fashioned oats
½ cup wheat germ
½ cup ground flaxseed
½ cup almonds
½ cup pecans
¾ cup dried fruit (I use golden raisins, pineapple, apricots, and cranberries)

½ tsp ground cinnamon
½ tsp salt
2 eggs
¼ cup honey
1 tsp vanilla extract
¼ cup shredded coconut (optional)
¼ cup mini semi-sweet chocolate chips (optional)

Directions

1. Preheat oven to 350°F. Grease an 8x8-inch baking dish with nonstick cooking spray.
2. Place the oats, wheat germ, flaxseed, almonds, pecans, dried fruit, cinnamon, and salt in a food processor and pulse until the mixture is finely chopped.
3. Mix together the eggs, honey, and vanilla in a large bowl until well blended. Add the oat mixture from the food processer along with coconut and chocolate chips, if using, and stir to combine.
4. Spread the mixture evenly into the greased dish. Bake 18 to 20 minutes, or until the edges turn golden brown. Let the mixture cool completely in the pan before slicing into bars.

Source: Adapted from No Whine with Dinner Cookbook[1]

53

Chicken, Farro, and Veggie Skillet

When you're meal planning, it's important to balance proteins, starches, and vegetables and this recipe meets all three criteria. Whenever I make a recipe that contains starches and vegetables, I always adapt it by tripling the veggies, because in my opinion, you can never have too many. This dish is fantastic whether served hot or cold, meaning it's great for dinner and perfect for leftovers the next day at lunch.

Makes 6 servings

Ingredients

For the Skillet
- 1 cup farro
- Chicken broth (optional)
- 1 lb. chicken tenders, cut into bite size pieces
- 2 large carrots, cut into 1" pieces
- 2 cups green beans, cut into 1" pieces
- 1 cup asparagus, cut into 1" pieces
- 6 scallions, thinly sliced

For the Sauce
- ¼ cup extra-virgin olive oil
- 2 TBS dried marjoram
- ½ tsp Kosher salt
- ¼ cup white wine vinegar
- 2 large shallots, diced
- 2 tsp Dijon mustard

Directions

1. In medium saucepan, cook farro in water (or chicken broth) according to package directions. Drain and let cool.

2. Using a nonstick skillet over medium-high heat, cook chicken, about 8 to 10 minutes or until cooked through.

3. In pot of boiling water, add carrots. Boil for 9 minutes. When there is 5 minutes remaining, add green beans and asparagus and boil until crisp-tender. Drain vegetables in a colander and rinse under cold water to cool.

4. In a large bowl combine farro, chicken, and vegetables. Add the sliced scallions.

5. In a small bowl whisk together the oil, marjoram, salt, vinegar, shallots, and mustard.

6. Pour the dressing over the farro, chicken and vegetables. Season to taste with salt and pepper.

Source: Adapted from Wellness Concepts[2]

lesson 5

Prioritizing Your Most Precious Gift

"You always have time for the things you put first."
—Unknown

Time is a gift and we have the choice whether to spend it wisely or foolishly. Everyone is given the same amount of time in a day. How we choose to spend it determines our productivity, but also our satisfaction levels. In my practice, I have had the privilege of meeting tons of great people. Some of those people are driven and motivated while others are just trying to keep up, because their lives revolve around putting out fires. How we choose to spend our time dictates our moods and our output.

Health is not just a state of being. We have to put in the effort. Life will always be there to throw us the unexpected. That is not a cliché; it is a cold-hard fact. We have to create an extra margin of time to allow for the unexpected if we want to stay on track and ultimately reach our goals. Placing boundaries around time creates a strong foundation. It doesn't come easy nor does it happen overnight, but eventually, it weaves into how we approach other goals in the future.

I often say, if the only thing I get accomplished is reading my Bible and exercising, it will be a good day. Both practices bring forth peace, stress management, and motivation. We're trying to improve our levels of health, fitness, and stress so we can live long, productive lives with the people we care most about. I want to be active with my grandchildren. Because my biggest motivation is being there for my family, it's important to make time for them, not only in the present, but also for the future.

nourish

Thanksgiving to Go

Our journey at Lehigh Valley Hospital was nothing short of an emotional roller coaster. Born just shy of 31 weeks, the girls spent their first six weeks of life at a level one NICU center about an hour away from our house. We knew they would come early given my history of deliveries. When I was pregnant with Jake, I went into labor around 32 weeks. The culprit to the premature labor, they thought, was dehydration. I was given a round of steroids just in case he decided to make his appearance early and delivered him at 37 weeks. Because he had the steroids five weeks earlier, he was born healthy and thriving. He would be the only child I brought home from the hospital the day I was discharged.

As a result of the early labor, my doctor sent me to a perinatologist, who did extensive testing. They couldn't find anything wrong and told me it shouldn't happen again. Parker was born at 38 weeks, but had trouble breathing after delivery. After observing him for an hour without change to his condition, the nurses told me he needed some extra help with oxygen due to lung prematurity.

After Parker was born, Jim went home to sleep. The drive to our house from the hospital was about 45 minutes. He had no sooner pulled in our driveway when I called him, hysterical, telling him he needed to drive an hour to another hospital to meet the ambulance, because the small community hospital where I delivered wasn't equipped with any level NICU and Parker wasn't responding to treatment.

Thankfully my mom was already at the house watching Jake, so Jim hopped in the car and drove in the middle of the night to be with Parker. Parker spent six days in the NICU and came home Halloween night, meeting his brother for the first time, who was dressed as a chicken.

Since no one could put a finger on my early deliveries, I was sent to a different perinatologist when I was pregnant the third time. I was followed closely by both my new specialists and my obstetrician and was told, yet again, that nothing was wrong and another early delivery was unlikely.

When I went into labor at 36 weeks, four days before Christmas, we knew I was heading for the same outcome. At this point in time, our small community hospital had a level two NICU and would be more prepared to help, if needed. Ben arrived the same day and spent the next two weeks at this hospital in the NICU. Despite spending most of the day on Christmas Eve at the hospital, we made it to church that night. I made it through one Christmas song before bursting into tears, telling Jim we needed to go back to the hospital. What kind of parents just leave their child all alone on Christmas Eve? Patient as ever, Jim was familiar with postpartum hormones, and we ended up making the 45-minute drive back to the hospital for the second time in one day.

Déjà Vu

Given my past three experiences, I was prepared to dismiss any and all doctors' prognoses about early labor not happening again. With my history and the fact that there were two of them, I knew, without a doubt, it would indeed happen again.

The girls were born nine weeks early and definitely needed the expertise of a level one NICU. The girls were able to get amazing care right from the beginning since we decided to bypass the small community hospital and planned their delivery at Lehigh Valley.

As anyone who has had a child in the NICU knows, the days are long and grueling. All you do is stare at the monitor … All. Day. Long. You try to will your child into getting better faster, but time is the only thing that helps. You try to be logical, but the fear and the hormones take over and you cry … a lot … well, at least I did. Never did I imagine that the short stays of my younger two boys would be preparing me for the scariest moment in my life.

When the girls were in the NICU, my days were split. I would get the boys ready for school in the morning, drive an hour to the hospital, stay with the girls from about nine to five, drive home from the hospital, and then be with my boys the rest of the night. I did this every day for six weeks.

Thankful for Good Health and Family

One particular day, Parker had a Thanksgiving feast at his preschool. I normally would have been at the hospital in the middle of the day, but we thought it was best for me to spend time with Parker, as he was looking forward to me being there. I got to the preschool and was waiting for the kids to come into the auditorium when my phone rang. It was the hospital.

I immediately thought "Wow, the girls must be doing great! Maybe they are thinking of discharging early."

The news I was expecting faded fast as I unexpectedly heard the doctor's

57

voice on the other end of the phone. My heart sank.

Bella was sick. They didn't know what was wrong, but she needed a blood transfusion immediately. Therefore, I had to give verbal consent over the phone right away.

I felt like I was on delay. Did I hear him right? This can't be happening. No, Bella was just fine yesterday. She was a little congested, but the nurse said she was fine. I don't understand!

I gave consent and immediately burst into tears. The preschool director, who happens to be my friend, walked by, noticing my hysteria. When she told me to go to the hospital, I felt this deep, gut-wrenching feeling that I needed to be there for Parker since I had missed so much of his life the past few weeks. It sounds ridiculous now, but at the time, I had no idea what to do. I decided to stay for the first 10 minutes to watch Parker walk over to my table. I gave him a big hug and told him how much I loved him, but that I had to go see his sister.

Surprisingly, he didn't look disappointed at all, so I rushed out of the building to make the drive to the NICU. On the way, I called Jim, and he decided to leave work and meet me there. I don't remember actually driving to the hospital. God was watching over me and all the other cars driving around me that day.

Jim was already there when I arrived and the doctors had started the transfusion. We were told the first couple hours were critical. Bella's heart stopped twice throughout the process. She eventually stabilized, and I stayed the night while Jim tended to the boys at home.

Exhausted physically, mentally, and emotionally, I had nothing left to give to anyone at that point. My eyes were so dry and swollen from crying, I could barely see. All I could do was pray for my sweet, little, baby girl.

I think I blocked most of my remaining time at the NICU out of my memory bank, but I do remember sitting on the glider in Bella's isolation room rocking back and forth. I must have fallen asleep for a little bit, because I remember waking up to the most beautiful sound. What was it? After a minute, I realized it was the graceful melody of the Doxology, sung by another mother to her own child. She had the voice of an angel. I would come to learn the next day her daughter, Miracle, was born at a little over 20 weeks. Her nervous system was so premature that even the touch of a human hand set her alarms off.

Here was a woman who was forced down a scary road, but through it all, was praising God's name through worship, and here I was, rocking on a glider, begging God not to let my daughter die. The moment was surreal and even as

58

I write these words to paper, I still get emotional.

Bella improved over the next 24 hours. She was diagnosed with rhino-virus (also known as the common cold) and her care team was able to meet her medical needs. Another week went by and the girls progressed to holding their temperatures, feeding, and overall thriving.

Charley came home the Monday before Thanksgiving and Bella was sched-uled to come home a few days after—Thanksgiving Day. The nurse asked us to arrive at 3 p.m. to sign her out. We made plans to grab Thanksgiving din-ner at Wegmans (a grocery story native to the Mid-Atlantic and Northeast region of America), since I was obviously not cooking.

All six of us arrived at the hospital on time. Jim stayed in the car with 22-month-old Ben and newborn Charley while I took Jake and Parker with me to grab Bella and all of her things. Jim and the babies couldn't get too comfortable, though, as our stay at NICU would be extended yet again.

I found out there was a slight problem with Bella's paperwork and we couldn't take her home just yet. An hour later, I was told no one had written her discharge papers and that finding a doctor on a holiday to write them up was going to take some time. Remember, the girl had been in the NICU for six weeks with significant events; this was not a quick note to write!

The nurses put all six of us in a private room and we proceeded to wait almost three hours for the paperwork to be completed. The nurse who told me to arrive at 3 p.m. made frequent visits to our room, in tears, constantly apologizing for ruining our Thanksgiving.

I can equate the last leg of this race to running a marathon. At this point, we have put in our 26 miles, but still needed to log in those last two-tenths of a mile to officially say we finished. We left the hospital a little after 8 p.m., hungry and tired. It was too late to order from Wegmans, so we found a diner and ordered four Thanksgiving meals to go.

By the time we finally reached our home, everyone was ready to eat. Of course, the girls woke up hungry, just as I was putting the food on the table. That year, we ate turkey and stuffing out of Styrofoam containers, holding crying infants, and it was the best holiday we've had to date. Our family of seven was finally all together the way it was meant to be.

My favorite healthy holiday tip is to always make the day about the people instead of the meal. This was one example where that tip couldn't be more poignant.

Planning holiday meals and tasting different dishes is part of the fun, but what if we invested the same amount of time into the people sitting around the table as we put into preparing the food? This past Thanksgiving, my dad took the time to write everyone around the table a note about why he was thankful for them. I still have my note in my purse for moments when I need encouragement. Another family tradition my friends use to celebrate Thanksgiving is using the same sheet as a tablecloth year after year. No matter where they go or who hosts, they bring the sheet for all who sit around the table to trace their hand. Then, in the empty space of every finger, they write the five things they were thankful for that year. I can't help but reflect on how special it must be to review the multitudes of hands traced year after year, watching how they grew in size and remembering what was important to every person at that particular time in their lives.

I encourage you to celebrate and create memories with the people around your dining room table. Set the phones down and look people in the eye. Thank God for the moments that only family and good friends can bring. Don't let everyday moments like eating dinner become a missed opportunity to let others know how you feel about them.

eat

'I Don't Know How You Do It'

One Saturday, Jake had a lacrosse game early in the morning. It didn't make sense for the whole family to come, so I offered to go with him, secretly enjoying the opportunity to sit by myself and actually watch the game. I rarely talk to other parents at games, partly because I'm introverted, but mostly because I'm playing referee to the four other children that really don't want to be there.

We arrived early enough for the team warm up, so I grabbed my blanket and proceeded to find a spot along the sideline. After settling in, I chatted with two moms about the boys' team and exchanged small talk about our sons' ages, homeroom teachers, and lacrosse positions.

One mom noted she hadn't talked to me before and I explained it was usually because I was trying to protect the crowds from my family's chaos. It's not unusual for people to look at me like I have three heads when I reveal how many children I have. I don't even notice it anymore. I realize large families aren't the norm, but it was always a dream of mine.

My friends think I'm a nutcase, but my inspiration for a large family was the movie, A Very Brady Christmas (cheesy, I know). I loved the idea of all the kids coming home for the holidays when they were all grown up, filling both my house and my heart.

The conversation somehow moved to cooking dinner at night and what kind of meals I prepare.

"How on Earth do you cook dinner every night?" one of the women said in amazement. "I have absolutely no time to cook, so we end up going through the Chick-fil-A drive-thru several times a week."

She continued to list out all of the extracurricular activities in which her three children were involved—all during one sports season!

In response to her original question, I smiled at her, "It's easy! We say 'no.'"

Having five kids is amazing, but it's expensive and time consuming, so it limits the number of things we can do.

My motto is, "I won't do for one what I'm not willing to do for all."

Those limitations end up working in our favor, because we don't become overscheduled. If all of my kids were in three different activities at the same time, I would be running through the Chick-fil-A drive-thru too, probably screaming at my kids the entire time! That's why I don't place judgment on this mom—she is doing the best she can, but she is still making a choice. Having her multiple children in multiple sports takes time and energy. Something has to give, and in this case, it's preparing a healthy dinner.

I get it—getting caught up in giving our kids every opportunity is an easy choice. We want our kids to be well rounded and explore multiple opportunities. However, there is also something to be said for cooking a healthy dinner every night. This choice teaches our children that taking care of our bodies is also important and necessary. It also teaches them not to run around and overextend themselves.

Too often, I see patients in my office who don't know how to cook. We are passing this trait down to our children every time we choose takeout. Remember, when you dine out, you will consume more calories, more fat, more sugar, and more sodium, mostly because you get larger quantities and because of the preparation methods. We are not doing our families any favors by choosing this route, unless we're trying to win a popularity contest with them, which is another topic for another book.

Nutrition takes time and energy—two items that are already in limited supply. That's what makes nutrition no small task. If you are overscheduled, trying to add healthy nutrition and exercise habits into the mix is doomed to fail. If you want to eat better, you also have to carve time out to cook. That may require you saying "no" to other opportunities. If you want to exercise, you have to make time to move your body. This may require you to wake up earlier in the morning, meaning you need to go to bed earlier in the evening.

Ten Minutes or Less

Just once I would like for someone to walk into my office and ask me for a recipe that takes two hours to prepare. I would imagine the request would go something like this:

"Adrianne, do you have any recipes that take a long time to cook? I'm looking to really extract and develop the flavors from each ingredient. My goal is for my family and I to all sit together at the table for approximately one hour or more, not only to enjoy the food prepared, but to enjoy each other's company, as well. Do you have a recipe for that?"

I can tell you right now that this will never happen, because no one has the time. Sure, we have all of this time-saving technology that supposedly makes our lives easier, but does it? I believe the only thing technology has accomplished is making our lives busier. I always chuckle when my retired patients ask me for quick recipes. Where do you have to be that warrants the need for dinner to be quick? You're retired!

The bottom line is that we are all too busy and that our busyness comes at a cost. Our bodies suffer physically when we run out of time to take care of them properly. Filling up on quick convenience foods and living a more sedentary lifestyle, because, "There is just not enough time in my day to cook or fit in a 10-minute walk," will leave us nutrient depleted, exhausted, and most likely, a few pounds heavier. The stress involved in trying to be five places at the same time (let alone remembering everything we have to do at each venue) wears on our mental and emotional health. Busyness has never been, and will never be, a good thing.

The Secret Solution

I'm going to let you in on a little secret that society either doesn't want you to know, or is too distracted to figure out on its own. No one will tell you this, but I will ...

If you can't put a meal on the table at night, you're too busy.

Food is a basic need. We all need food to survive; therefore, it should be somewhat of a priority. If Chick-fil-A is a weekly need versus a once-in-a-while treat, then that is a problem. Society will tell you to keep up with the Joneses. I will tell you the truth ... don't.

Forget the health implications for a minute and let's just look at what we are teaching the little people around us. I'll paint the picture: it is now perfectly acceptable for a family to scarf down its meals while in a moving vehicle. You may even try to justify it with, "just this once," knowing full well it happens on a regular basis. Over time, this lifestyle has solidified into the core essence of your family. Even more discouraging, your children accept this fast pace as normal.

Sounds a bit absurd when you read it that way, doesn't it?

One of my patients, the mother of two active boys, struggles with finding the time to make dinner for her family. Both boys play for different travel baseball teams, which means driving to and from practices throughout the week and traveling to different cities on weekends for games and tournaments. Her justification for all of the takeout meals was that it was only for the short term. She went on to explain that in four weeks, when the season was over, things would settle down and making dinner at home would be much easier. However, after three weeks of downtime the chaos would begin again with the start of football preseason.

"So let me get this straight," I started. "You have three weeks off in an entire year where things settle down and then you'll be able to make dinner?"

"Actually, I have four weeks off if you count Christmas break," she remembered.

"Oh, well then that's okay. I was thinking you only have three weeks off out of 52. Four weeks is perfectly acceptable."

Could you sense the strong hint of sarcasm in the air? Imagine being in the room with us!

Our culture will pressure us into thinking we should give our kids every single experience possible, every day, multiple times a day.

I will tell you the truth. This is not okay. Our kids need us to be present, not stressed-out chauffeurs. Our kids need to feel heard and have real, live conversations, looking into our eyes, seated around a table; not talked to from the rear-view mirror in between bites of French fries.

When I was growing up, my parents took us to a babysitter named Esther over the summer. Both of my parents worked and I loved spending the day with her and the other 20 kids she was watching. Esther wasn't overwhelmed at all. She loved kids and spent time with each one of us. Get this: she always made us a hot lunch ... from scratch! Could you imagine that happening today? That's hard to do when everyone is looking for quick, easy recipe ideas. Despite her level of competence, years later, the state shut Esther's operation down once it became privy to how many kids she was watching.

People always say to me, with amazement in their eyes, "I don't know how you do it with five kids."

My reply is always the same.

"I think five kids is easier."

It's impossible to do everything for each kid. If I can't do it for all five, then I don't do it for any of them. Logistically, it doesn't even make sense to get five kids to five different practices. My husband and I alternate who works nights so there's only one person to get everyone everywhere. Eating a meal together is really important to us, so if that can't happen, then we reevaluate our activities.

Listen, I get how easy it is to get sucked into it all. One summer, we did the travel lacrosse thing and we were miserable. All of us!

I'm not here to judge anyone, because if it works for you, then great! Professionally, though, I'm seeing too many people struggle; so, I'm giving you permission to say "no." Choosing not to be busy is extremely hard and counter cultural, but it's also a gift. Just like summers are a gift to teachers, less busyness is a gift to families. Ask anyone about his or her favorite childhood memory. More often than not, the response will be a family dinner, likely at his or her grandparents' house. My guess is grandma didn't make a meal that could be assembled and consumed in 10 minutes or less.

When it comes down to it, we all have a choice. One of my most favorite quotes, which I repeat to myself often, comes from Thomas Monson. He says, "Choose the harder right instead of the easier wrong."

How can you apply that wisdom in your own life? Perhaps it's saying "no" to another obligation and saying "yes" to your health and your family's well-being.

repeat

Evacuate the Masses!

It was approximately five years ago when one of the members of my family took it upon himself to evacuate an entire building of people with one simple move. I will give you three guesses as to which family member that was, but you should only need one if you've been paying attention.

You guessed it. It was Ben!

The memory of that night is so very vivid. Ben was three, the girls were about one year old, Jake was seven, and Parker was six. It was a beautiful spring evening. My parents came to visit so we could all go to our elementary school's art show. We were meeting my mother-in-law and sister-in-law at the school. The plan was to walk the halls together, admiring the artistic gifts that the children had to offer.

Everyone was smiling, taking pictures, and laughing. Including my parents and in-laws, we had six adults and five kids—two of them strapped into a stroller. It's important to note that we had a proper adult-to-child ratio going in there.

I can't even say I remember the moment Ben ran ahead of us, but it was as if he had it planned out from the beginning. There wasn't any time to yell, "Stop," "Don't," or, "No!" It all just happened so fast. My three-year-old ran right up to the fire alarm and just pulled. Immediately the alarms started sounding and the lights began to flash.

Jim rushed over to the alarm to try to push the bar back up, but apparently it doesn't work that way and he was unsuccessful, much to our disappointment. Looking around, I saw people moving toward the exits. Jim began to walk down the hall again to admire more artwork.

"Jim, you need to go tell someone our kid did this," I reasoned. "People are beginning to evacuate!"

We had no choice but to follow the crowds. The next thing we know, we were standing outside, waiting for the fire trucks to arrive. I found the school nurse also waiting outside with her family and told her it was Ben who caused the scene. A couple seconds later, the principal drove up to the entrance. She was at the event earlier, but had gone home for the evening. She asked us if we knew the name of the child who had caused all of this commotion. Luckily, the school nurse was a friend of mine and she withheld from ratting me out on the spot. Meanwhile, I hid amongst the crowd of confused art show attendees.

Once the school was deemed safe, the families began filing back into the school for a second attempt at a fun, leisurely evening. I felt like I couldn't breathe. As a safeguard against further embarrassment, I forced Ben to hold one of our hands the entire duration of the evening. For two years following that incident, I had extreme anxiety walking the halls of the art show, paranoid for a repeat performance. I'm happy to report it was Ben's first and only offense.

Expect the Unexpected

The unexpected will happen. As much as we try to prepare and plan, life doesn't always work out our way. I had a better-than-one-to-one, adult-to-child ratio that night and I still couldn't keep my kid from evacuating an entire building of people.

It's important to be able to have some flexibility, knowing that life may throw you a few curveballs. Diets are one of those things that need flexibility, as well. If you approach your intake as something that needs to be rigid, structured, and unwavering, then you are setting yourself up for failure.

Health comes in all forms and is constantly in flux. Rarely do I find someone killing it on all 3 matrices (physical, emotional, and mental), but rather, it's a constant ebb and flow based on factors like environment, other people, and circumstance. The more rigid you try to be with your diet, the more upset you will become when things don't go as planned.

Now, don't get me wrong … I love a good plan. I drive Jim nuts on vacation when I ask him what he wants to eat for dinner while he's preparing his breakfast. He's always on me to relax and just take it one thing at a time, but that's not how I operate. A good plan allows me to know when I can take a risk and when I need to pull back.

At the end of the day, a plan is a set of ideals. If they work out—great! If not, evaluate. Could you have changed the outcome? If the answer is no, then there is no need to deliberate and stress. I teach my patients a phrase I learned from one of my mentors, Michele Francis (she actually heard this theory at a LEARN program she did for weight control, hosted by weight management guru Kelly Browmell):

"Do not let a lapse become a relapse become a collapse."

A lapse will happen every now and again, so acknowledge it and just move on. See the one-time occurrence for what it is, make a change if possible, and move forward. The more expectations you put on others to adhere to your plan, the more likely you will be disappointed if and when things move in a different direction.

What areas in your own life do you need to add flexibility? Do you try to follow a bunch of rules with your diet or exercise routine, driving everyone around you crazy?

Choose a day this week and skip your workout and see what happens (I promise you, it will be okay). Allow yourself to share an ice cream with your kids tonight and notice the looks on their faces. Do you follow a strict schedule at home that leaves no room for downtime or free play? Just like we are wired for action, we are also wired for rest. Take a look at your schedule right now and insert a time block to do absolutely nothing. Force your body to relax by breathing and just existing in the present. There are plenty of progressive relaxation apps out there that can be of great help to you here.

What areas in your day-to-day life could benefit from a few boundaries? I used to think that I was great at creating boundaries, but the more I'm learning about myself, the more I'm realizing that I'm absolutely terrible at this. In my attempt to "do it all," I overcommit and then stress out about how I'm going to accomplish everything, which leaves me depleted and anxious. When we try to do it all ourselves, we rob others of utilizing their gifts.

What responsibilities can you delegate to others? Which committees can you let someone else take over? Where can you be a supportive resource rather than being the source of action?

The great news about finding answers to these questions is that you are your best source of knowledge and there are no hard rules, nor is there a one-size-fits-all approach. Usually, the best way to tell if you need more balance is to observe how others act when they are around you. If everyone is jumpy and on edge because they're afraid you'll lash out at them if the plan is disrupted, then it's time to re-evaluate the plan. If you find yourself getting too regimented, evaluate your routine so you can add more spontaneity. You may just find yourself laughing and enjoying life a little more when you add in some fun. Your overall health will benefit when you incorporate more excitement in your life!

choose your plan

Affirmation

Repeat this statement every day this week:

"Choose the harder right instead of the easier wrong."

Action

Say "no" to the drive-thru this week and opt to prepare meals at home. If it's easier, prep all five days the weekend prior to save time during the week. Bonus points if you prepare a meal that takes longer than 10 minutes.

Achieve

Be fully present at mealtime, meaning all electronic devices (including the TV) need to find another home away from the dinner table. Think of one way you can express gratitude to the people you are eating with at your next meal.

Analyze

How can you say "no" to another responsibility and "yes" to your health and well-being this week? What tasks can you delegate? Write these out in your journal.

Accountability

Answer the below questions in your dedicated healthy lifestyle journal:

What change did you attempt to make this week?

Were you happy with the results?

What challenges did you encounter?

How would you do things differently next time?

5-star recipes
Salmon Cakes with Lime Yogurt Sauce

It can be a challenge to prepare something quick, tasty, and healthy on a night. I save even more time by using the salmon pouches from the grocer to skip the step of draining the juices from a can. Fish is a great source of and heart-healthy omega-3 fats. The goal should be to eat fish twice per wee recipe will make it simple to achieve.

Makes 4 servings

Ingredients

For the Sauce
1 lime
½ cup light mayonnaise
½ cup plain Greek yogurt

For the Salmon Cakes
6 pouches (2.5 oz. each) sk
boneless pink salmon
½ cup red bell pepper, cho
½-1 small jalapeño, chopp
finely (optional)
¼ cup scallions with tops,
1 TBS fresh cilantro (can ;
fresh parsley or dill), chop
1 cup panko breadcrumbs
⅓ cup light mayonnaise
1 egg

Directions

1. To make the sauce, zest the lime into a small bowl. Combine z juice of the lime, mayonnaise, and yogurt, and mix well. Cover a in refrigerator.

2. For the salmon cakes, combine salmon, pepper, jalapeño (if usir lions, cilantro, breadcrumbs, mayonnaise, and egg until well incor

3. Divide salmon mixture into four even parts and form into pattie: nonstick skillet or grill pan over medium heat. Cook salmon cak minutes, or until golden brown. Gently turn over cake and cook tional 4 minutes.

4. Top salmon cakes with dollop of lime sauce.

Source: Adapted from It's Good for You (Pampered Chef)[1]

Sweet Potato Black Bean Chili with Avocado

If you're looking for a great twist to chili, look no further! Like all good chili recipes, this one takes some time for the flavors to develop. Slow cookers are great for cutting corners without sacrificing flavor. Steps 1 through 3 can be prepped over the weekend and then cooked in your slow cooker when you're ready to enjoy.

Makes 4 servings

Ingredients

2 TBS olive oil
1 medium yellow onion, chopped
2 red bell peppers, chopped
3-4 sweet potatoes, peeled and chopped into ½-inch cubes
4 garlic cloves, minced
1 TBS chili powder
1 tsp ground cumin
¼ tsp ground cinnamon
1 bay leaf
2 cans (15 oz. each) black beans, rinsed and drained
1 small can (14 oz.) diced tomatoes, including the liquid
2 cups chicken broth
2 avocados, diced
12–15 blue corn tortilla chips, smashed
Chopped fresh cilantro or parsley for garnish

Directions

.. In a large stockpot, add the oil, onion, bell pepper, and sweet potatoes and cook over medium heat. Stir occasionally, until the onions are soft and turn translucent.

. Turn the heat down to medium-low and add the garlic, chili powder, cumin, and cinnamon. Cook, stirring constantly, until fragrant, about 30 seconds.

. Add the bay leaf, black beans, tomatoes with their juices, and broth. Transfer to a slow cooker, turn heat to low, and cook for 4 to 6 hours, until vegetables are tender and liquid has reduced. Remove the bay leaf.

. Serve chili in bowls, topped with diced avocado and tortilla chips. Garnish with fresh cilantro or parsley.

lesson 6

Body Basics

"Self-care is giving the world the best of you, instead of what's left of you."
—Katie Reed

As busy women, we have become pros at taking care of others. Thirteen years ago, I attended a "Women of Faith" conference. Robin McGraw (Phil McGraw's wife) was the guest speaker. That evening, she attributed her mom's lack of self-care to her ultimate death. Robin's mother was so busy taking care of everyone else that she forgot to take the time to take care of herself. That lecture was a moment of clarity. I finally realized the importance of making myself a priority and no longer saw the concept of self-care as a buzzword or fantasy. Now, it is a mandatory practice I want to include into my very core.

My kids' elementary school teaches the concept of bucket dippers and bucket fillers. The premise is to be a bucket filler for others by using kind words and deeds instead of depleting a person's bucket with harsh words and actions. Self-care is totally a bucket-filler move. If we want to fill our neighbors' buckets, we cannot pour from an empty cup. We can no longer rely on or expect other people to fill our buckets for us, so we have to take initiative and fill our own each day.

Fill your bucket by building a solid nutritional foundation. Water is an essential nutrient for our bodies. Omit it and everything else suffers. The simplicity of drinking enough water might seem too small of a concept to have that big of an impact, but my experience will teach you otherwise.

Finally, knowing what health habits take your body to a state of wellness reinforces your foundation. Becoming aware of our struggles is always the first step to lasting change.

nourish

Feeling Like a Mama Pig

Have you ever visited a farm? We are fortunate to live near a wildlife center that rehabilitates animals and is open to the public as a park. It's not a very large establishment—I would estimate 20 or 30 animals total—and it takes roughly 20 minutes to walk through. This is the perfect amount of time to accommodate the short attention spans of small children and toddlers, and you can turn it into an afternoon excursion by packing lunches and eating at one of the picnic tables near the river that borders the farm.

In addition to rehabilitated animals, the park used to have a farm section. One of our family's favorite parts of the trip was looking at the baby pigs. I remember feeling bad for the mama pigs, because they had eight to ten babies jostling for position to feed all day long. The mama would just lie on her side, resigned to the fact that this was her job for the day and she wasn't going to get much else accomplished.

I only had the boys when this area was open to the public, so I could only empathize with her a little in the breastfeeding department. I was one of those ladies blessed by God with an abundant milk supply. My friends and I always joked that I could feed a small village and that my purpose in life may be to become a wet nurse. For all the breastfeeding mamas out there, you know how hard, draining, and dehydrating breastfeeding is. Those babies literally suck the life right out of you.

Then, God decided to have a sense of humor and gave us twins. When we got over that shock and started talking logistics, I began thinking about what that could look like with nursing. I was already determined to breastfeed, because I knew supply would not be a factor. I started reading everything I could get my hands on for information how to feed two. Did I dare even try to feed them both at the same time? Let's just say that was a hard "no" when they were newborns. It wasn't until they were closer to six or seven months and they could help themselves get into position that I was successful feeding them both simultaneously.

The very first time I tried, the image of the pig flashed through my mind almost immediately. I wasn't feeding eight or ten, but I was maxed out with two and it was the most odd, confusing, and weird sensation that I have ever experienced.

Nursing two babies (separately or together) was a new level of draining.

I was so tired. There were many days I got nothing done. I would lay on the sofa, resigned to the fact that this was my job for the day and I wasn't going to get much else accomplished. Those babies sucked the life right out of me and I felt like there was nothing I could do to replenish or refuel.

You may not be breastfeeding but how close does this story resonate in your own life when it comes to feeling drained? Are you running around exhausted, giving your time and energy to those around you, resigned to the fact that this is just how it's going to be? Do the words "self-care" make you chuckle and think "that's a luxury only rich, kid-free, or retired people can experience"?

Self-care is one of the most important things you can do for yourself and your family. At work, I have patients fill out a self-care worksheet identifying areas where they are doing well and those where they need to pay more attention. Once we identify strengths and weaknesses, we map out a plan for change.

When it comes to weight management—or anything you're trying to accomplish—it's important to, first and foremost, take care of yourself. Nutrition and exercise take time and energy, which is why so many people are unsuccessful. Most people are already burning both ends of the candle when they try to add weight loss to their to-do lists.

You can already guess that their successes will be short lived. In order to be successful, you have to set yourself up for success. You have to do the things that put you in a position to master your goals. One of those necessary things is self-care. I like to view self-care as a choice. I choose to take care of myself so I can take care of others well. I can choose discipline and go to bed at a time that makes me feel energized the next day, or I can choose to stay up late and watch my favorite TV show, which will leave me feeling depleted and cranky. Either way, I choose.

What does self-care look like to you? For some it could look like going to bed earlier or setting boundaries with family and/or coworkers. For others, it could look like seeking therapy when needed or carving out time to spend with a good friend. Further, it could look like turning the TV off or saying no to that 10th volunteer opportunity for which you know you'd be the perfect candidate.

It could mean viewing workouts like non-negotiable doctor appointments or letting yourself cry instead of holding it all together. The good news is that you don't have to do all of these things at once. Just pick one area that could use a little more love and start there. Being kind to your body shows self-respect, but it also models to others to do the same. If you're a parent, your kids are watching you and how you choose to do life. If you're running around exhausted, your kids will think that this is normal and continue in your footsteps.

Imagine who you could be if you took the time to invest in you. My guess is you would be unstoppable!

eat

Twins, Life Vests, and Port-o-potties

You know exactly where this story is going if you have ever taken a small child inside a port-o-potty. I'll see your cringe and raise the stakes by adding in a second child. I'll raise the stakes higher when I tell you both children were girls, and I will even take that to an unprecedented height by adding that both girls were wearing life vests.

Nobody in his or her right mind wants to use a port-o-potty, but in this particular story, we had no other option. We decided to take all the kids on a family-friendly, white water rafting trip. The girls were five, so that tells you how fast the rapids were. Think more of a family float with miniature rapids along the way. Because the water was lower than normal, the plan was for the bus to drop us off at our lunch spot first, and then we would proceed down the river for the remainder of the afternoon.

As we were enjoying our lunches, Jim and I made sure to remind everyone to drink a lot of water. Being the peak of the day, the sun was directly overhead without a cloud in sight; we didn't want anyone to get dehydrated.

Then, seemingly out of nowhere, the guide announced we would be leaving in five minutes, to which the girls, on cue, announced they both had to go potty. Apparently, we weren't the only ones to come up with this earth-shattering idea, because the line was already long by the time we walked over to the facilities.

I won't even go into the smell or the visual of what we witnessed inside those tight quarters. People were going to the bathroom as quickly as possible so they didn't miss the ride.

Let me preface this by explaining that it is not physically possible for two five-year-old kids to use the bathroom fast. Young girls are not wired that way. I don't remember who went first, but I do remember making the one who waited stand as still as possible, with her hands in the air, until it was her turn. I used the mom voice, threatening that if she as much as tried to touch anything, I would not let her go rafting.

Meanwhile, trying to hold the other girl up over the potty so she didn't touch the seat, I began to feel a bit wet—yes, she peed all over my arms. I could hardly breathe, because it smelled so bad and her life vest was covering up my mouth, forcing me to use my nose to breathe.

It was so hot and so tight inside that bathroom, and to top it all off, I could hear people mumbling outside wanting us to hurry up. Didn't they know how hard this was?!

I felt deserving of a prestigious award for being able to pull the first girl's shorts up without knocking the other one over or falling over myself. But wait ... I had to do all of this nonsense all over again with twin number two!

Sweating profusely and holding my breath in long bursts, I pulled myself together with a short pep talk and proceeded to go through the whole drill with my other daughter, all the while making sure the first didn't touch anything. I can't recall what there was more of—urine running down my arms or tears being contentiously held in because of it. Did I mention the life vests were making an already impossible circumstance 10 times harder?

We finally finished up, able to escape that insanely small, incredibly smelly and oppressive hot box. I started to walk down the path with the girls and some other rafters when I realized I had a big piece of toilet paper stuck to the bottom of my shoe. Of course I did! Jim was nowhere to be found, but I was convinced he was enjoying a cocktail somewhere on a cruise ship with the boys. When I finally caught up to him later, he reported that he went ahead because he was trying to get us a good raft. How sweet and helpful.

Hydration is King

Okay, so yes, I just shared with you the most horrific memory of taking a double urine bath in a port-o-potty, and now I am going to tell you how important it is to stay hydrated throughout the day and to be vigilant about your own potty breaks. Experts tell us we should pee around six times per day and that our urine should be clear and copious (meaning a lot).

A good rule of thumb is to take your current body weight and divide by two. That's how many ounces of water you should drink daily. Caffeinated beverages, such as soda, teas, and coffee can act as a diuretic, so I personally don't count these toward the total goal because I want people to get in the habit of drinking more water.

Fruits and vegetables can contain large quantities of water, so, if you're choosing these as the base of your diet in addition to your water bottle, you're likely getting enough. A lot of people don't care for the taste of water, so feel free to add your own flavors by infusing it with citrus, berries, cucumber, or mint. I promise you this: the more you drink regular water, the more your body will crave it and come to appreciate the flavor.

Another good rule of thumb is to try to drink most of your water by the early evening. I don't recommend playing catch up on the water you missed that day starting at 9 p.m. Good sleep is so important and hard to come by for some, so let's not make that more difficult by getting up multiple times per night to use the bathroom.

Proper hydration is so important for our bodies to work optimally. It gives us better mental clarity, performance, energy, and stamina. Our bodies work more efficiently when hydrated too. More times than not, we mistake thirst for hunger and end up consuming unnecessary calories. If you have ever found yourself in front of an open refrigerator trying to figure out what you want, that is not hunger. Typically, that is thirst. The more hydrated you are, the easier it is to discern true hunger from thirst.

When I begin to work with a new patient, our first goal is always to drink more water. One trick is to get a water bottle with a straw, since most people tend to drink more this way. Remember, water always through a straw, alcohol never through a straw (for the same reason). Carry your water bottle with you everywhere. You're more likely to drink if you have it nearby.

Finally, always be sure to hydrate properly before a rafting trip. You wouldn't want to get dehydrated being out in the direct sun for hours on end. You may even be able to tell a funny story about it someday!

repeat

Aren't I Too Young for That?

Some people are highly allergic to poison ivy. I am one of those people. If I stand within 10 feet of the plant, it seems like I get it. If I wash the clothes of people who touched it, I get it. I have been on steroids multiple times to control it, taken countless oatmeal baths, and heck, one time I just made oatmeal and poured it all over my arms! Living on a farm surrounded by woods is not a good place to live for someone who is highly allergic to poison ivy.

About three summers ago, I got poison on my arms from working outside. I just so happened to have a dermatologist appointment and said something to the doctor about a few red spots I was starting to see on my face. She told me I must have touched my face, because she was seeing signs of poison there too. We were leaving for my cousin's wedding in Virginia in a few days and I could just imagine my face breaking out in the itchy rash, leaving me miserable. The doctor offered me a steroid and I quickly obliged. I'm happy to report the steroids did their job and my face was clear and itch-free in time for our departure.

One week later, I must have been outside working, because I had poison on my arms again. I noticed the middle of my back was itchy too, but when I scratched it there, I felt some pretty intense pain. Because it was on my back and hard to see, I continuously asked Jim to look at it. He repeatedly said, "Looks like poison to me." So, I thought I must have been making the pain up in my head.

I also started to notice it hurt to sit against the back of a chair or lay on my back in bed. Every time I asked Jim to look at it, he would tell me it looked like poison. Next I noticed the rash and pain starting to spread to the side of my body. I figured I must have tried scratching my back and managed to rub the poison from my arm against my side. Great, not only were my back and side in pain, but I was losing my mind too!

Things took a different turn that Friday night when I was taking a shower and found a lump on the right side of my breast. Panicking, I screamed for Jim to come upstairs to see if he could confirm what I was feeling. After he did, I instantly began the process of planning my funeral. I told him it was important that he remarry for the kids. I also started thinking that there would be no photos of me at the viewing since I was the one who took all the family pictures. So, I made a mental note to plan a photo shoot so my kids would have a family picture to remember me.

It was Friday night, which meant I had to go through the whole weekend before being able to call a doctor. It was the worst weekend ever!

Monday was a century away, but when it came, I was quick to call my gynecologist, who subsequently referred me to a breast specialist who couldn't get me in until the end of the week. Since I had already gone through an entire weekend of funeral planning, I staunchly refused to wait one more day.

Thankfully, after some desperate begging, I was able to convince my family doctor to fit me in the same day. The doctor began the examination and looked at me, slightly confused.

"Adrianne, I really don't think the lump is in the breast tissue," he said. "It feels more like your lymph nodes. Are you sure you're not sick or fighting a cold?"

I didn't know whether to be concerned or relieved. I told him I felt fine, no sickness at all, but did have some poison on my arms. After further examination, he confirmed the poison, but shook his head, explaining that wouldn't typically activate my lymphatic system in that way. He continued to ask me questions about potential symptoms, but every time, the answer was "no."

That was when it hit me: the poison on my back and side! Since it was the only lead we had for the moment, the doctor asked me to pull my shirt up in the back to show him. Almost immediately, he had the diagnosis.

"Adrianne, you don't have poison on your back, you have shingles!" he chuckled. "Doesn't it hurt?"

Wait a minute, **what**? I have shingles?! The first words that come out of my mouth were, "Aren't I too young for that?"

He told me anyone can get shingles if they have had the chickenpox virus. Further investigation led us to believe that the most likely cause was the steroid prescription I had taken the week prior. Apparently, it can wake up the virus in your body.

I couldn't wait to tell Jim that I wasn't crazy for thinking my poison rash was painful. All this time he said it was poison and here I had shingles! Oh yeah, and I probably should tell him I'm not dying and to cancel the photographer.

Long story short, the doctor gave me medicine that I ended up being allergic to, so I had to wait it out and let the virus run its course. It's amazing what a little perspective can do for your pain tolerance. I never knew a 35-year-old could get shingles. Now, I think twice before asking for a steroid for poison ivy.

The fact is we're not too young to get any disease even though we may feel invincible. The Centers for Disease Control (CDC) announced in 2013 that, at this point in time, more than half of all adults have at least one chronic disease.[1] To me, that translates into the idea that young adults are acquiring chronic diseases that were historically only seen in aging populations. I can confirm that statistic, because I see young adults coming to my office for help to control their blood sugars, blood pressures, and high cholesterols. Because of these statistics, the CDC went on to identify the top five health behaviors that can put someone on the path toward health, or at least minimize the risk for contracting a disease. The behaviors are:

1. Maintain a healthy weight
2. Practice consistent exercise
3. Do not smoke
4. Moderate alcohol intake
5. Get enough sleep every night

The recommendations are reasonable. In fact, they are all basic principles that we instinctively do for our kids, especially when they are at young age: we feed them balanced meals, sign them up for activities, enforce bed times, and prohibit them from ingesting toxic materials. Notice, it doesn't say you must run a marathon every year or never drink alcohol. It doesn't say you have to have a BMI of 20 either. The only one that is an absolute is the smoking recommendation, because there is no gray area when it comes to cigarettes.

These are general, healthy behaviors that anyone can adopt, yet only 6.3 percent of Americans are meeting all five criteria.[2] Yes, you read that right: 6.3 percent!

That statistic is heartbreaking and sad. There are no other words to describe it. I realize everyone has his or her vice(s). Some people are really good at eating well and exercising, but drink too much on the weekends. Other people may be able to check off the first four behaviors, but in order to do so, miss out on key hours of sleep at night.

It's easy to justify, or come up with excuses as to why we can't accomplish all five, but the reality of it is this: not following these guidelines puts us on the path toward disease. If we're not adhering to these basic principles, then we are putting our bodies at risk for disease. If we are aware of, but do not apply these principles, we can no longer claim ignorance, blame genetics or deny our own responsibility when our blood pressures are running high. Unfortunately, we are not too young for disease, as the research confirms.

So, what one area can you start to improve from the basic list of five? Do you need to decline that extra drink on the weekends or perhaps go to bed earlier? Can you start preparing more vegetables with dinner or find a friend to be your walking partner after work? Pick one thing to start today. Together, let's change the 6.3 percent for the better!

choose your plan

Affirmation

Repeat this statement every day this week:

"I choose to join the 6.3 percent."

Action

Divide your current weight in half to approximate how many ounces of water you should consume every day.

Invest in a nice water bottle with a straw to help you reach that goal.

Achieve

This week, make a conscious effort to engage in one form of self-care. Think about how you may be lacking in certain areas of taking care of your mind, body, and soul and pick one area on which to focus.

Analyze

Which one of the five recommendations outlined by the CDC do you struggle with the most and what is one step you can take to create change?

Write it down in your journal and make an effort to initiate that change in your daily life.

Accountability

Answer the below questions in your dedicated healthy lifestyle journal:

What change did you attempt to make this week?

Were you happy with the results?

What challenges did you encounter?

How would you do things differently next time?

5-star recipes

Burrito Salad Bowl with Creamy Avocado Sauce

I first made this dish in an effort to eat more vegetarian meals and be more conscious about our environment. I was surprised all five kids gave this recipe the thumbs up and I have been working it into our rotation ever since. Of course, if you prefer to add more protein, feel free to add grilled chicken, shrimp, or fish.

Makes 4 to 6 servings

Ingredients

For the Sauce
- 1 ripe avocado
- 5 TBS water
- ½ cup cilantro leaves
- 3 TBS lime juice
- 1 clove garlic, minced
- 2 TBS plain Greek yogurt
- ¼ tsp salt
- Black pepper to taste

For the Bowl
- 1½ cups frozen corn
- 1 TBS olive oil
- 1 red onion, peeled and chopped finely
- 1 tsp ground cumin
- ½ tsp salt
- 2 (15 oz.) cans black beans, rinsed and drained
- 1 cup brown or wild rice
- 2 cups vegetable broth
- 4–6 cups shredded romaine lettuce
- Pico de Gallo (can also use salsa)

Directions

1. Add avocado, water, cilantro, lime juice, garlic, yogurt, ¼ tsp salt and pepper into a food processor or blender. Blend until smooth and then transfer sauce to a small bowl.

2. In a nonstick skillet, add the frozen corn and ¼ cup water and cook over medium heat. Reduce heat to low and keep warm for later.

3. Add oil, onion, cumin, and ½ tsp salt to medium sauce pan and cook over medium heat. Stir occasionally until onions are translucent, about 5 minutes.

4. Stir in beans, rice, and broth and bring to a simmer. Cover, reduce the heat to low, and cook for 15 minutes, until the liquid is absorbed.

5. Divide the romaine lettuce and rice mixture evenly among serving bowls. Top each bowl with corn and Pico de Gallo. Drizzle creamy avocado sauce on top and serve.

Source: Adapted from The Complete Cookbook for Young Chefs[3]

Peanut Butter Banana Ice Cream

Sometimes self-care means treating yourself to something sweet. Our family enjoys eating a sweet treat over the weekend, and this recipe finds its way into the rotation often. This lightened-up version is a great alternative to ice cream and a great way to use up ripe bananas (instead of making banana bread).

Makes 2 to 4 servings

Ingredients

2 ripe bananas (the browner the banana, the sweeter the ice cream)
¼ cup smooth all-natural peanut butter
½ TBS coconut oil
½ tsp ground cinnamon
½ tsp vanilla
Kosher salt

Directions

1. Slice the bananas and lay them flat in a single layer on a cookie sheet. Place bananas in the freezer for at least 2 hours.
2. When ready to mix, take the bananas out of the freezer and let them sit for 4 to 5 minutes out on the counter.
3. Place the frozen bananas, peanut butter, coconut oil, cinnamon, vanilla, and pinch of kosher salt in a blender and puree until creamy and smooth.

Source: Adapted from Food Swings Cookbook[4]

lesson 7

Mind-Blowing Lessons
You Never Learned in School

"Mindfulness isn't difficult, we just need to remember to do it."[1]
—Sharon Salzberg

Whenever my husband decides to run a yellow light or make a sharp turn, he exclaims to the kids, "Hold on to your girdle, Myrtle!" Well, that is how I feel about the next five lessons. Strap on your seatbelt, because I'm about to take you on a ride!

How you eat has as much of an impact on your health and weight as what you eat and how much you eat. Only once I started becoming conscious of my eating style and habits was I able to make radical changes to my overall health. The beauty of developing habits is that you are ultimately training your brain to help your body react and respond to new encounters.

As you will soon come to see, I am all about consistency. There are always going to be times in your life when you make the unhealthy choice—it happens. However, if you are in the consistent habit of eating in a way that speaks mindfulness, your portion sizes will decrease and the guilt you previously felt whenever "cheating" will be virtually nonexistent. You will make purposeful decisions, which will make you feel proud and confident. Who knew that following five simple, practical steps could reduce—if not eliminate—unnecessary, mindless stress eating and ultimately change the course of your eating style forever?

Oh, and one more thing ... make sure you're sitting down to read this lesson.

nourish

Indoor Picnic Table

About four years ago, we were sitting around our dining room table one Saturday afternoon eating lunch as a family. As you can imagine, a large family eating lunch (or any meal for that matter, let's be honest) always produces a huge mess. The table and floor are a disaster and sometimes the walls get in on the action. One time, Jim found broccoli hidden in an antique metal pot sitting on the side table. The real treat is finding moldy food in a corner. Jim always said there is no reason to get a pet, because we live with animals.

At the time of this particular meal, we had a dining room table utilizing two or three extender leaves. Jim bought it for $25 at a moving sale down the road and we felt like we hit the jackpot. The only problem with a table that has leaves (and seven people gathered around it) is that food would frequently get stuck in the cracks between them. After every meal, we would have to pull the table apart to clean it, which normally turned into a once a week job, since we only had enough energy to do so that frequently.

It was a pain, but our alternative to purchase a new table just wasn't in the budget. After lunch, Jim decided to pull the table apart to clean it. Once he started pulling and saw the mess we needed to clean up, I heard him mutter, "Forget it," and then watched him begin to disassemble the table.

I started to question what he was doing, but he didn't say a word; he just continued pulling apart the table until it was in pieces small enough to get out the door. The next thing I know, he had his keys in hand and walked outside. I ran after him, but by the time I caught up, he was already backing out of the driveway. My confused look prompted him to tell me that he would be right back.

It's not like Jim to storm out of the house or leave us for any extended amount of time in anger, so I was thoroughly confused about what just happened. I didn't have time to dwell on it, though, because I had my own list of things to do. I yelled for him to take a kid or two wherever he was heading and then proceeded back inside to wash the dishes.

An hour later, I heard Jim's car roll into the driveway. I was folding laundry in the back room when I heard this thud coming from the dining room followed by a screeching sound as he unlocked the legs to a folding table.

That's right, the love of my life just brought home a Costco-brand, outdoor picnic table, complete with attached benches, and he was smiling from ear to ear.

"The best part about this table is if it gets too dirty, we can just fold it up and hose it down outside. Isn't this great?"

I'm sorry, what just happened? No, this is not great. You just disassembled and threw out our perfectly good, wooden, normal table and replaced it with an outdoor, industrial picnic table. This had to be a joke. This was only temporary, right? Please say we are going to the furniture store next week to replace this plastic table!

I bet you'll never guess what our dining room table looked like four years later … If you guessed the Costco picnic table, you're a winner! In Jim's defense, it really did wipe down nicely and we didn't have the chore of cleaning in between leaves any longer. It had become our story for so long that I didn't even notice its oddity. That is, until someone new came to visit and did a double take when she saw the table. Oh, that's right, yes, you are seeing that correctly. That is an outdoor picnic table with a tablecloth on top. Don't ask. Let's just all pretend it's normal.

We have a lot of great memories around that table. This is where we hosted holiday meals and birthdays. If you thought crowding around a small table was difficult over the holidays, I challenge you to try it with a picnic table. Not only did everyone have to eat with the same hand (sorry left handers), it also required a level of fitness to get in and out of the table for those sitting in the middle. We had successfully put 10 people around the table even when the kids weren't so little anymore. Want to see how much your family likes each other? Buy a picnic table and it will tell you.

Our table also holds memories of homework, storytelling, and tears. It is where our family gets together to share our successes and our failures. The rooms in our old farmhouse are small and segregated. There is no option to watch TV from the dining room table, which means we are forced to look and listen to one another when eating. There are no distractions.

I can't urge you enough to move dinner away from the TV and move cell phones into another room so they are out of sight and out of mind. From a nutrition standpoint, we tend to eat more when there are screens to distract us. We tend not to remember the experience of eating because of distraction. Psychologically, we want to repeat that behavior since we missed out on the experience the first time.

More importantly than weight management, we miss out on the amazing gift of time with others. We get to learn about each other and have an opportunity to let others know they are loved—that their words are important and valued. Always remember that the most important part of your dining room table is the people sitting around it, not the material it's made from or its shape.

It's also important to note that in order to value the people around the table well, we must sit there long enough to engage in real, honest conversation. Did you ever notice that people tend to sit longer during a holiday meal? They linger at the table instead of being in a rush to get to the next thing, which allows for conversations and relationships to develop.

Instead of asking children how their days were, which is a perfectly acceptable question (but is often met with a one-word response), go a little deeper and ask, "What was the funniest thing you saw or did?" or "Did you notice anyone acting quiet today?" or even further, "How did you show someone kindness today?"

Meals are great opportunities to teach our children appropriate table manners and how to become more observant of the people around them. Taking the time to listen to their responses allows you to help them navigate their way. Aim to sit down at your table, together as a family, for at least 20 minutes during a meal and watch your relationships move to a new level.

We finally did find a new dining room table at another moving sale. We had four beautiful years with that picnic table, but our growing kids made it difficult to all fit around it, especially with grandparents and extended family at the holidays. As funny as it sounds, I am forever thankful for the life lessons an outdoor Costco picnic table taught me.

eat

Sit Down to Eat

It was a week after Halloween and I was in the mood for a little piece of chocolate. I strategically made my husband go through the candy when the kids got home from trick-or-treating so I wouldn't know what candy they brought into the house. Once I know what is there, it's all over—I'm going to want it.

I had placed the newly filled bucket of candy high in the soffit above the stove so it was inconvenient for "the kids" (also known as me) to get to. That afternoon, though, I was feeling stressed, or bored, or maybe a combination of the two, and I wanted something sweet to eat.

I quietly climbed onto a chair so as to not alert the kids to what I was doing and found a miniature pack of M&Ms. That would do it! I tore open the package and dumped the candy into my hands when all of a sudden, I heard footsteps pattering toward the kitchen. Panicked, I did the only thing any rational person in my situation would have done; I shoved all of the candy into my mouth and pretended I was cleaning something.

The kids arrived, and lucky for me, asked me a simple question. I was able to simply nod, both answering and dismissing them simultaneously. I would be lying if I said I wasn't a little annoyed at them for interrupting my experience, so, to make up for it, I climbed back on the chair to grab another piece of candy and enjoyed that one in peace.

There are so many things wrong with this situation that go beyond me stealing candy from my kids. I committed multiple violations in the mindful eating department. Mindful eating involves paying attention to what is going into your body. It means you are fully present, focusing on how food tastes and the emotions you're feeling while you are eating it.

Mindful eating is intentional. I wish I could take credit for putting this montage of advice together, but the credit goes to clinical psychologist Dr. Susan Albers,[2] who specializes in eating issues, weight loss, body image concerns, and mindfulness. I have been following her work for years and using it to help hundreds of patients. I have added my own little spin on some of these helpful tips along the way.

Be Engaged With Your Meal

All of these mindful eating tips begin with the letter S. The first S stands for **sit down to eat**. I'm going to take the liberty and add **at a table, from a plate**. This is a *big* one and probably the one I personally struggled with the most.

Do you sit down when you eat? Every time? Or do you find yourself standing at the counter inhaling your food? Do you eat hovering over the kitchen sink? Perhaps you quickly stuff M&M's into your mouth, hiding the fact that you are eating them from family members like I did.

Whatever your situation, sitting down to eat from a plate speaks intention. It says, "I'm engaged in what I'm doing and am not going to be distracted by what is going on around me."

At our house, we have a peninsula in our kitchen with two stools. It is a rare occasion I get to sit down on one of those stools since they are always occupied by a child, so I used to find it just easier to eat my meal standing up on the other side, ready to get condiments, drinks, or extra utensils someone else may need. It was a bad habit I had developed and often led me to overeating because of all the distractions. I wasn't fully enjoying my meal, because of all the interruptions. More times than not, I ate faster when I was standing.

One morning, Jim made himself an egg sandwich and I watched him stand over the counter to eat it. When I suggested he sit down, he replied, "Why? I'll be done eating in 30 seconds." That's exactly the point I was trying to make!

Another bad habit I had developed was eating at the counter while standing up when I arrived home at night after work. Since I tend to work more evenings, I get home late and am hungry. I would tell myself, "I'm only going to eat a few bites of leftover dinner, so why bother going through the work of sitting down and getting a plate?" Before I knew it, those first few bites would show me how hungry I really was and I would start to inhale the food. Putting the food on a plate and sitting down has guaranteed that I am more intentional about the volume I'm consuming.

Think of it this way: for those of you with kids, I want you to think about a time when you were at a family member's or friend's house for a party. Your four-year-old comes up to you and says he's hungry. Now, you know he must be really hungry, because four-year-olds would always rather play than eat. You fix him a plate and then usher him over to the table to start eating so he doesn't make a mess on your host's floors. At the first sign of fullness, he gets up from the table and goes back to playing with the other kids.

Now, I want you to think about your own eating habits. You're at a party and all the food is sitting out on a table. Everyone is socializing and snacking from the buffet. You mindlessly grab two pretzel sticks and start munching. Before you know it, you have lost count and have no clue how many you have eaten. Was it 8 or 28 pretzel sticks? Who knows, because you're not paying attention!

If you had to go get a plate to put a few pretzel sticks on it and then find a table to sit, away from your friends (like you did for your four-year-old), you may find that those two pretzel sticks don't seem very important anymore. First, you may realize you're not even hungry, and second, you don't want to miss out on the conversation. Sitting down and eating from a plate means you're committed to the task at hand. Sitting down and eating from a plate speaks mindfulness and will set you up for success.

By shoving M&M's into my mouth while I was standing up, I missed out on the chance to really enjoy the chocolate I was craving. If I had sat down and ate from a plate, I would have enjoyed the experience the first time without having to call a mulligan with the second package.

This tip is extremely powerful, yet easily dismissed. If you're not doing this already, I urge you to start. If you forget, just sit down as soon as you remember, even if you only have two bites left. Instead of telling yourself you'll remember next time, change the behavior right away. Chances are, if you try to remember the next time, you'll forget again.

Athletes experience something similar here. My high school track coach would yell at me to stop shuffling my feet when I ran. Do you think he said, "Adrianne, at practice tomorrow, I want you to remember to pick up your feet higher"? Heck no! He said, "Go back to the start line and do it again the right way." It only took me a few times to remember to pick up my feet, because all those extra laps were exhausting.

The same applies to you. Every time you eat, sit down at a table and eat from a plate. If you forget to practice your new habit from the beginning, self-correct as soon as you catch yourself standing up. I promise you, it's a habit worth creating.

repeat
We Are That Family

I am an introvert. That may surprise a lot of people, but it's true! Nothing causes me more angst than a room full of strangers. I tend to find comfort in the nearest wall, hoping someone will come find and engage me. I realize for work it's important to network, but it literally petrifies me. I'm good for the introduction part, but then my mind goes to mush. I cannot think of a single educated thing to say. My mind defaults to the weather **every time**. There's only so many times you can talk about the sun, rain, and temperature in a conversation before it turns weird. I know this from experience.

After the first meeting I attended for our youth's high school ministry program as a new volunteer, I was told to go out to the lobby and mingle with the kids prior to the service starting. It just so happened that prom was the previous evening, so I was told it should be easy to strike up a conversation. Well, it's only easy if you like talking to strangers.

I was fortunate enough to shadow our children's pastor, who had no problem getting in there and creating dialogue. She did everything possible to work me in the conversation and I could hold my own for all of about 30 seconds.

My three default questions were: "Did you have fun last night? Can I see a picture of your dress? ... and, "Did you get stuck in the rain?" I know—more weather questions!

After that, the conversation would get quiet, and I couldn't think of anything else to say. I kid you not, I almost asked one young girl what she ate for breakfast that morning. What can I say? I panicked!

I'm definitely much more in my element when I'm in my counseling room at work. I find it easy to connect with people on a more individualized basis and can find ways to keep the conversation flowing. In all honesty, food is an easy topic. Everyone eats and everyone has an opinion of what a healthy diet looks like. I can usually throw out a fact or study and it can drive our conversation for the duration of the appointment. I also love public speaking and feed off the energy in the room. Put me in a meet-and-greet environment, though, and you'll find me along a wall talking about the weather.

Because I'm an introvert, I struggle with the kids' sports scene. A lot of the parents congregate together, laughing and sharing stories along the sidelines. Since I find it challenging to start up a conversation, I tend to sit by myself. I also sit by myself, because I'm trying to control my tribe from annoying others and robbing them from a serene experience. Small children do not enjoy sitting for an hour along the sideline watching their brothers or sisters running around the bases or up and down a field. They want to run, fight, play, scream, and make noise. When the girls were really little, I felt like we were a traveling circus, always putting on a show for the bystanders—a loud, boisterous act for viewers to enjoy, pointing and laughing the entire time.

Trying to Keep the Peace

It was a smolderingly hot day and the field on which Jake was playing lacrosse had no shade in sight. It was as if we were stranded in the middle of a desert. We brought our small tent as a means of shade since Jim is emphatic about sun protection. I'm pretty sure the tent was made for one person, but we figured out how to cram six people in that thing.

It didn't take long for the heat and close quarters to start messing with everyone. Since the girls were so little, Jim and I were each doing our best to hold a squirming lump of heat on our laps, drenched in our own sweat.

The two younger boys were fighting in the back of the tent, causing the top of the tent to bend backward, exposing us to more direct sunlight. I can only imagine what we looked like from a distance; probably a circus inside of a miniature tent. At one point, Jim told the kids to reapply more sunscreen. Parker picked up the can and accidentally sprayed some on Bella's face. She immediately screamed like a banshee. We only brought so much water with us, and were trying to ration it for drinking, but I used it to clear any sunscreen from running into her eyes.

Wrestling a two-year-old in 99-degree weather was impossible. Jim told me I needed to take her to the emergency room just in case she got sunscreen in her eyes. I disagreed and said her crying was a good thing, because it was flushing the sunscreen out for her.

We continued to argue in our miniature tent. The heat was rising to what felt like 120°F. After a few minutes, Bella started to calm down and she eventually fell asleep, most likely exhausted from all of the crying.

As I held her, I noticed her body was like a blanket on mine, but at least she was not crying anymore. Jim had also significantly calmed down as he was trying to keep cool, holding a toddler of his own.

We made it through the third quarter of Jake's game in peace when all of a sudden, I felt warmer than usual ... wetter than usual. Ugh! Bella just peed all over me.

Trying to complain to Jim was a moot point. His solution was for me to deal with it and not wake her up. Yes, we are *that* family—the ones trying to keep our peace so you can enjoy yours.

Habits, Not Goals

Whether we are trying to keep the peace or engage in a conversation, how we are wired can push us toward success or keep us in the grips of fear. Our personality types can help or harm us in certain situations. Many people deal with their emotions through food, using it as a coping mechanism or form of reward.

As much as I teach mindfulness, I also must teach that mindful eating is a muscle. You have to train it just like you would train you body for a sporting event. You cannot simply will yourself to eat differently, just like you can't will yourself to react differently in certain situations. It takes practice.

Professional basketball players aren't great at foul shots just because they woke up one day and said, "I want to be good on the free throw line." No, they practice thousands of free throws each season, trying to get it right, so that on game day they can just show up and execute.

If you want to change your habits, you need to practice change. Then, you need to repeat your new behavior(s) over and over until you can run on autopilot.

Rather than making goals, make habits. Habits are huge when it comes to our lifestyles, because they are a form of pre-deciding how you will respond to a situation. If you are in a habit of drinking low-fat milk, you avoid the precious time of deliberating which product to buy in the dairy aisle. There is not a decision to be made, because you know exactly what you want. That's the freedom of creating a habit! No deliberation in the moment. You just do what needs to be done.

If I ever want to get away from that wall in a room full of people or talk to other parents at sporting events, I need to practice engaging in conversations in those types of environments. In the same way, if you want to be more engaged with your meal, you need to practice sitting down at every meal.

Thank goodness health is not a competition, but rather a journey. Eventually you and I will get to our destinations in our own ways, on our own timelines, but not without practice.

Think of a habit you would like to change or add right now and visualize yourself doing it in your mind (close your eyes and do this now). Take special note of your actions, your surroundings, and your attitude. Are you confident in your actions? Are there other people around you, or are you by yourself? What other circumstances are occurring simultaneously when you are engaging in this new habit?

Once you have it in your mind how this will play out, I want you to do it. For example, put your fork down in between each bite, put on your sneakers and walk into the gym, or walk right past the snack food aisle at the grocery store without going down the lane. The next day, do it again. The day after that, do it again. Consciously practice your habit until you don't even think about it anymore and it just becomes a part of your essence. Whether it takes 21 days or 60 days, it doesn't matter. Just keep moving forward. Just keep practicing.

choose your plan

Affirmation

Repeat this statement every day this week:

"I will be mindful when I eat."

Action

Every time you eat something, including bites, licks, and tastes, sit down at a table and eat that item from a plate.

Achieve

This week, focus on asking the people around your table open-ended questions (see examples from this lesson) to spark quality conversations and learn more about each other in the process.

Analyze

Identify one habit you want to change. Pause a moment and visualize yourself engaging in this new habit.

Write out an action plan for following through on it. Make sure you write down, in your journal, any anticipated roadblocks and how you will overcome them. Then, go out and do it!

Accountability

Answer the below questions in your dedicated healthy lifestyle journal:

What change did you attempt to make this week?

Were you happy with the results?

What challenges did you encounter?

How would you do things differently next time?

5-star recipes

Easy-to-Remember Turkey Sausage Soup

*Because sitting down to eat is a non-negotiable at our house, I sometimes need to create quick meals that are easy to consume. This patient recommendation is perfect for busy weeknights when my kids have practice and is so easy to memorize since you only need one of everything. My kids are **big** fans, and other patients I have shared it with love it too!*

Makes 4 servings

Ingredients

1 lb. bulk turkey sausage
1 tsp dried Italian seasoning
1 (14.5 oz.) can diced tomatoes
1 (32 oz.) container low-sodium chicken stock
1 cup orzo
1 bag spinach
1 handful shredded Parmesan cheese
Basil

Directions

1. Brown the turkey sausage in a stockpot. Drain any fat from the pan when it is finished cooking.
2. Add dried seasoning, tomatoes, and chicken stock. Bring to boil.
3. Once the mixture is boiling, add the orzo. Cook according to package instructions (about 6 to 8 minutes).
4. Turn the heat down to medium low. Add spinach, Parmesan cheese, and basil (fresh or dried is fine) to taste. Stir until spinach is wilted. Serve immediately.

Spinach Turkey Meatballs

This is one of my favorite recipes. I love it for its simplicity, taste, and because it feeds the army sitting around my dining room table. I always sneak one or two, fresh out of the oven, because I can be impatient waiting for the rest of the family to meet me for dinner.

Makes 8 servings

Ingredients

1 (10 oz.) box frozen chopped spinach, thawed
2½ pounds ground turkey
1 small onion, chopped
1 egg
4 garlic cloves, minced
¼ cup milk
¾ cup bread crumbs
½ cup parmesan cheese
¼ tsp dried thyme
½ tsp dried parsley
½ tsp dried oregano
¼ tsp crushed red pepper flakes (optional/adjustable)
Salt and Pepper
Olive oil for drizzling

Directions

1. Preheat the oven to 400°F.
2. Using clean kitchen towel, wring the spinach until most of the liquid has been removed.
3. Place the ground turkey in a large bowl. Add the spinach, onion, egg, garlic, milk, breadcrumbs, cheese, seasonings, and season with salt and pepper. Mix well.
4. Form into 24 meatballs and place on baking sheet. Drizzle with olive oil.
5. Roast for 20 to 25 minutes or until cooked through.

Source: Adapted from Rachael Ray[3]

lesson 8

Do as the Southerners Do

"Once she stopped rushing through life,
she was amazed how much more life she had time for."
—Unknown

In this section, we revisit the idea of slowing down. This time, we'll pay attention to the speed in which we eat. It seems like everything we do here in the Northeast has to be done fast. Unlike the slow pace of the South, speed is revered and celebrated, because there's always another project waiting in the wings. Utilizing time wisely, which includes multitasking, means accomplishing what most people would plan for a week to be accomplished in one or two days. There is this expectation of a quick turnaround and so the pressure yields more productivity—but at what cost? Unfortunately, the cost is either health or mental sanity. One must suffer in order to thrive in this fast-paced life.

Most of my work is helping individuals find balance to their chaotic schedules. I'm constantly looking for places where we can insert the word "and" instead of just "or" for both pleasure and quality of life. Can we eat quickly *and* have good health? I was on a mission to find out.

Then there's this issue of competition. The South may have taught me how to slow down my pace, but my competitive nature needed a good, honest assessment and evaluation. In my quest for the word "and," I needed to know if there was a way to be genuinely happy for my female counterparts or was I always going to view other ladies as competition? Let's go there. I'm not ashamed to say it, because I know I'm not the only person to ever have these thoughts. Remember, bringing ideas into the light also brings the ideas into a space of healing.

nourish

Hen House

My husband endearingly uses this expression often, describing the competition between women—that jockeying for position and the resulting jealousy, thereafter. It can happen in a place where women predominantly hold positions (eg. hair salons, PTA meetings), but really can occur anywhere.

The term "hen house" is derived quite literally, and I can attest to this because we own chickens, all of them being feisty women. There is a definite pecking order between them and if one goes down, the rest are there to pounce on her, peck her until she's bloody, and drive her to the bottom of the totem pole. We call our chickens "the ladies" not because of their sex, but because of their ruthless behaviors. Women can be fierce.

My best relationships are my girlfriends. Finding a good girlfriend is difficult. Despite our feistiness, what women need most are safe people with whom we can open ourselves up, be honest, and share life. This type of friendship is a treasured gift.

There was a Similac commercial years ago, which depicted the many stereotypes of different moms. You had the working moms, the stay-at-home moms, the breastfeeding moms, the bottle-feeding moms, the exercise moms, the only-make-your-own-food moms, the PTA moms … each of them fighting for their passionate causes. We get so caught up in defending our ways, proving why our way is superior, we forget the one thing we have in common: we're all moms just trying to do our best.

I am not at all proud of my hen-house moment. I was working with another woman entrepreneur from a similar industry and we were trying to see if our businesses could complement one another. We planned an event and created guidelines for each of us to use in order to ensure a successful outing. Unfortunately, some of the terms were not met, so I canceled. The other business owner wanted to continue moving forward, but for me, it wasn't a good fit at that time.

She challenged my business ethics, which left me extremely defensive. Feelings were hurt, communication was muddled, and disappointment arose from both sides. I take ownership for not picking up the phone and having an adult conversation, but the truth is, I'm not confrontational and I was scared. I created a dramatic scene in my head of what I wanted to say and got myself all worked up, which affected my mood and ultimately my family, for days.

I told a few of my closest friends what happened, looking for validation. What concerned me the most was why the situation made me so angry and fired up every time I thought about it. I like to think I'm rational three weeks out of the month, but this struck deeper. It took me a few weeks to realize what upset me most was when she challenged my ethics. I work hard to create a morally healthy work environment. It is extremely important to me, and probably to her as well, which is why this situation hurt so much for both of us.

Women can be cruel. We can spot a weakness and go for the jugular. On the flipside, we can also be great cheerleaders, listeners, and support for one another. We must always consciously choose the latter, even when it's not popular or if we simply don't want to do so.

Let's keep it real—women are constantly checking each other out from a body perspective, trying to figure out where they fit in. It's not a good feeling. I once had a patient who refused to go to a mother-son dance at school, because she didn't like the way she looked in a dress and therefore didn't want her peers to see her either. Her son begged her to go, told her to wear pants, but she wasn't comfortable enough to go to the dance. That story intensely tugged at my heartstrings. This woman's insecurities kept her from experiencing a special moment with her son!

I want to lead the charge for us all to agree, right now, to stop checking each other out and instead celebrate our differences. Let's stop calculating how many people we are thinner than/bigger than and enjoy the dance. Unfriend/unfollow the people you follow on social media who project inferiority. Stop looking at the accounts that show unrealistic body images and make you feel bad about your own body. I've had to do it, despite trying to tell myself that I was keeping it for motivation. Deep down, I was trying to shame myself into trying harder. Some days, it would lead to overeating on perceived forbidden foods, because I couldn't measure up.

Health is **never** a competition! Every single one of us is on our own journey and it is **never** okay to push your agenda on someone else without his or her permission or without being asked your opinion, first. Choose to be a cheerleader! Build up instead of tear down. Life is hard enough without adding unnecessary competition to the mix.

I'm grateful for the situation that arose with my fellow female business owner, because it was an important teaching moment. It's not about who is the most ethical, successful businesswoman; it's about celebrating two women who are doing their very best.

The same goes with your women coworkers, friends, and acquaintances.

Imagine how many lives could be enriched and changed for the better if we rallied behind one another and supported each other. We can choose not to be a hen house and peck each other bloody. Instead of being jealous, we can be thankful for the women killing it and showing us the possibility that more exists. We can choose to build up and be genuinely happy for each other's successes.

eat
Slow Down, Partner

Last year, our family went to Tennessee for our summer vacation. Jim and I had visited the Smoky Mountains before kids and always thought it would be a fun place to revisit someday. Our family loves to be outdoors, so we planned our trip to include plenty of hiking and sightseeing.

Living in the Northeast, we have become so accustomed to the fast-paced lifestyle and impatient population that it just feels normal. When we visited the South, we were exposed to a much slower pace of living. People held doors for us and we noticed no one was in a rush to get anywhere. Cars rarely drove over the speed limit, and everyone paused to take the time to exchange greetings with us. Even more impressive—they waited to hear our responses! Here in Pennsylvania, it's nothing to ask someone how he or she is doing while moving forward and missing the response. In Tennessee, it felt as if no one had an agenda, which was extremely odd in comparison to our life in the suburbs of Philadelphia. It was exciting and refreshing to experience and our family immediately gravitated to the culture. If the goal of vacations is for time to slow down, we found it in the Smoky Mountains of Tennessee.

Channel Your Fullness Signal

I can't help but find the resemblance between slowing down the pace of life and slowing down the pace of eating. Both require intention and both elicit a more positive, gratifying experience. I graduated high school in a class of 170 students, so we had the luxury of playing multiple sports each season and making each team. The only downside was fitting in all of the practices, which typically meant taking five minutes to eat dinner. This habit continued to follow me well into my collegiate and early adulthood years.

One morning, as I downed a bowl of cereal, I caught myself strategically placing the next bite next to my mouth; ready to shovel it in the moment there was adequate space. How silly was it to be eating so fast considering I didn't have anywhere to be? I'm not proud of being a naturally fast eater, because it led to overeating.

It takes 20 minutes for the fullness signal to travel from your stomach to your brain. The problem with eating your meal too fast is your brain doesn't have all the information it needs to make an informed decision about whether or not your body is still hungry. Have you ever gone into a restaurant **starving** only to leave feeling sick and stuffed? The body goes from one extreme to the other without any warning signs when you eat too fast.

To prevent speed eating, divide your plate into four quadrants and try to take five minutes to eat the food inside each quadrant. If you find that difficult and finish in under 20 minutes, stay seated for the remaining time in order to allow the signal time to catch up with your brain.

Eating quickly is a common mistake most of my patients engage in. It takes a lot of practice to slow down. We are social creatures, so it's easy for us to mimic the speed of the people around us. I met one patient who told me he eats fast because of his time serving in the Navy, even though he hadn't served actively in 30 years. I told him it's time to come up with a new excuse.

Eating slowly will help your digestion and ability to listen to your body's cues for fullness. It will also enhance your satisfaction with the meal, itself. You will enjoy your food when you take the time to taste it. Remember, your taste buds are on your tongue, so be sure to allow the food to spend more time there than in your stomach. Focus on extracting every ounce of flavor from your meal. Eating slower will also help you to remember eating the meal, a mindful practice where you are present and engaged with the experience. Often, many of my patients eat mindlessly, leading to the consumption of excess calories and a desire to repeat the behavior, because they don't remember doing it the first time.

We can all take a lesson from the residents of the Smoky Mountains and slow down. Get to know your neighbor, hold the door for someone, and enjoy a slow, relaxing meal together.

repeat
Evaluate Your Eating Speed

In our previous lesson about mindful eating, I was hiding from my kids in the kitchen, eating some M&M's, when they came around the corner out of nowhere. I quickly put all the candy in my mouth so I wouldn't get caught, missed out on the desired experience, and ended up eating more candy to make up for it. So that brings us to the second mindful eating tip: this time S stands for **slow down**.

How fast do you eat? Are you usually the first one done at the table or the last? I admit, I'm a fast eater, but am actively working on changing that habit. Usually running around, overscheduling, poor time management, or bad habits are to blame, but that doesn't mean I need to accept it.

It can be a natural human behavior to want to match the eating speed of those around us. You may not naturally be a fast eater, but if your family or coworkers are, you're at risk of becoming one too.

One night, the whole gang was enjoying an invigorating game of Dutch Blitz when one of the boys asked to open the tin of popcorn we got as a Christmas gift. You may be familiar with the large, metal tin, with three flavors of popcorn—cheese, butter, and caramel. We opened the lid and everyone dove in.

It didn't take long for the pace to speed up as everyone started to panic, thinking they may not get their favorite flavor. I started to realize I didn't even taste the popcorn after a little while. I was shoveling it in as fast as the kids just to keep up.

I decided to stop the madness and grabbed a paper towel to hold my handful of popcorn. Now I could control the speed at which I was eating, because I had all the popcorn I needed right in front of me, instead of keeping up with the crazies. I enjoyed those last few handfuls of popcorn much more than the bites I shoveled in at Mach speed.

Pause, Slow Down, Be Intentional

There are many practical ways to slow down your eating—chew each bite 25 times, put your fork down in between each bite, or eat with your non-dominant hand. Studies show eating with your non-dominant hand can slow you down at least 20 percent,[1] which is pretty impressive. When I shared this tip with a patient, she looked at me and said, "I'll never get the fork to my mouth, I'm not that coordinated! I'll be so frustrated with the process and may just give up on eating. Is that your plan?" I love that shear honesty!

Jena La Flamme, author of *Pleasurable Weight Loss*, explained in a webinar series that there are many highly complex systems in our bodies, working hard every second of the day and we have no control over them. We don't have to tell our hearts to beat or stomachs to digest food. We don't have to tell our lungs to expand and contract. Our bodies do all of this instinctively.[2]

Hunger and fullness are also instinctual. If we actually listen to our bodies, they will tell us when we are hungry and full. For example, think of an infant. The baby cries when he's hungry and turns his head away when he's full. There's no overthinking it. The complexity of humans goes beyond our instinctual side and adds another layer—our minds. This is what separates us from other mammals, but also gets us in trouble when it comes to eating.

When our minds get involved, we can engage in restrictive or binge-type behaviors, trying to adhere to a socially acceptable norm or rebelling against it all. A baby has no interest in being a certain weight, so he is able to listen to his body's signals. An adult living in a weight-conscious society doesn't have that same luxury. La Flamme challenges her clients to tune into their "inner mammal" before eating in order to stop this cycle. Sounds a bit quirky, but stay with me.

Before a meal, La Flamme advises to place your hand on your heart or your stomach. If you put your hand on your heart, feel your heartbeat. If you put your hand on your stomach, imagine the process of digestion, or feel your stomach rumble. Tune into one of your body's instinctual systems that you have absolutely no control over yet keeps you alive every day. Next, take five deep, cleansing breaths, taking the time to thank your body for not letting you down and make a decision to trust and honor the cues it gives you. Do not try to override hunger and fullness signals with what your mind thinks is best. Let your body guide your volume.

This stuff works because it's another opportunity to pause, slow down, and be intentional with your meals.

I try to be a little more discreet when channeling my inner mammal by placing my hands under the table and feeling my wrist for my pulse. As I feel my heartbeat, I immediately thank God for giving me a body that is instinctive and has kept me alive up until this point. I also remind myself to pay attention to the signals my body will give me during the meal.

Instead of five deep, cleansing breaths, I take two in order to avoid my food getting cold. While I'm breathing, I pray or listen to one of my other family members pray for the meal we are about to eat. It's calming and sets the tone for the pace of the meal. My stress level is low (for the moment) and I'm ready to eat in a calm, civilized manner.

Whether you are channeling your inner mammal or eating with your non-dominant hand, slowing down the pace of your eating is a helpful tool to creating a more mindful eating environment. The next time you catch yourself eating faster than normal, put your fork down and take a deep breath. Don't let the people you eat with dictate the speed at which you eat. Move

103

at your own pace, paying attention to the signals your body gives you. This advice can transcend into other areas of your life. Identify some moments in your day when you can slow down and thank God for the people around you. Never underestimate the gift of time or the power of gratitude.

choose your plan

Affirmation

Repeat this statement every day this week:

"I trust my body to tell me what it needs."

Action

Divide your plate into four quadrants. Take a minimum of five minutes to finish each quadrant. If you find this practice difficult, stay seated for at least twenty minutes before deciding if you need a second helping.

Achieve

Before each meal, take two to five deep, cleansing breaths to both calm and relax you before eating. This action will set the pace for your eating speed.

Analyze

Choose to be a cheerleader! How can you compliment or build up the females in your life? Identify ways to encourage others with positive words or actions.

Accountability

Answer the below questions in your dedicated healthy lifestyle journal:

What change did you attempt to make this week?

Were you happy with the results?

What challenges did you encounter?

How would you do things differently next time?

5-star recipes
Chicken Dumpling Soup

This is a family favorite and a dish that speaks thoughtfulness through its familiar flavors. I typically bring it to friends when they just had a baby, moved to another house, or are simply in need of some comfort food. If I'm cooking this for someone else, I always triple the batch so my family can enjoy it too.

Makes 4 servings

Ingredients

2 TBS olive oil
3 leeks, white and tender green parts split lengthwise and thinly sliced across
5 stalks celery with leafy tops, thinly sliced
2 large carrots, sliced thin
1 bay leaf
Salt and pepper, to taste
1–2 cloves garlic, minced
1 (32 oz.) container low-sodium chicken broth
2 cups milk
1 lb. chicken tenders, cut into bite size pieces
2 packages (approximately 35 oz.) gnocchi
1 cup chopped flat-leaf parsley

Directions

1. In a large soup pot or Dutch oven, heat the olive oil over medium heat. Add the leeks, celery, carrot, bay leaf, and salt and pepper, to taste, and cook until the vegetables are soft, about 10 minutes. Add garlic and cook 1 minute longer.
2. Add the chicken broth and bring to a boil. Stir in the milk, lower the heat and cook until the soup begins to simmer at the edges.
3. Add the chicken and gnocchi and cook for 5 minutes or until chicken is cooked through.
4. Remove the bay leaf and stir in the parsley. Serve immediately.

Source: Adapted from Rachael Ray[3]

Cheesesteak Stuffed Mushrooms

I made this recipe for the first time when the Eagles played in the Super Bowl (going for a Philly theme) and it got rave reviews from the crew. Using a fork to eat your cheesesteak always leads to a much slower eating experience.

Makes 4 servings

Ingredients

Nonstick cooking spray

8 oz. thin-sliced sirloin steaks

Salt and black pepper to taste

¾ cup onion, chopped

¾ cup red pepper, chopped

1–2 cloves garlic, minced

¼ cup plain Greek yogurt

2 TBS light mayonnaise

2 oz. Neufchatel cheese, softened

2 tsp Italian seasoning

4 oz. shredded mild mozzarella cheese

4 large Portobello mushroom caps

Directions

1. Preheat the oven to 400°F. Grease a baking sheet with nonstick cooking spray.

2. Gently scoop out the gills of the mushrooms and spray the tops with cooking spray. Season steak with salt and pepper.

3. In a large nonstick skillet add the steak. Cook over medium-high heat about 2 minutes on each side, until cooked through. Remove from pan and let rest for 5 minutes before slicing. Set aside.

4. Using same skillet, reduce the heat to medium-low, spray with cooking spray and sauté the onions and peppers for about 5 minutes, or until soft. Add garlic and sauté one minute longer.

5. Add the steak back into the pan along with the yogurt, mayonnaise, Neufchatel cheese, Italian seasoning and mozzarella cheese and stir to combine. Divide mixture evenly into the mushroom caps.

6. Bake in the oven until the cheese is melted and the mushrooms are tender, about 20 minutes.

Source: Adapted from Skinnytaste.com[4]

lesson 9

Keep It Simple

"I believe that a simple and unassuming manner of life is best for everyone, best both for the body and the mind."
—Albert Einstein

I like simple. I don't like knick-knacks, clutter, lawn ornaments, or papers and magazines. I either recycle or throw everything out. Now, you may be wondering, "But what about that adorable picture your kid made three years ago of the cute bunny that actually looks like a scary dragon?"

What about it? I don't even remember that existed. If I kept every single piece of artwork my children have ever created, there would be no place to sit or walk in my house. I'm already terrible at cleaning. I don't need more things to move and organize when I actually get motivated to do some housework.

Years ago, my mom drove over to my house with two big tubs of childhood memories. She handed them to me and said, "Here you go, I'm not storing these anymore." I was so upset—not because she handed them off, but because now I had to find a place to store them. They live in the barn, because there is no room left in the house. I would be surprised if the items are still intact.

Clutter is stress. I already live with six people that cause me stress at various times of the day. Simplifying our lives brings so much freedom. The same goes with how we approach our eating environments and how we decide to fill our mental space. Eating food while other distractions are present, or filling our days with social media, creates clutter for us to sift through. The amount of energy that takes can be too great a challenge to overcome. So, I invite you to walk with me to a land called freedom.

109

nourish

Does Facebook Cause Diabetes?

Clearly, this is not a documented scientific fact. Since nutrition is a science, we need repeated, double-blind, randomized studies that prove cold, hard facts. There have been no studies proving Facebook and diabetes relate to one other. I will argue there is a correlation.

One of my colleagues and friends, Erika, while studying for her Certified Diabetes Educator exam, told me that type 1 diabetes was up 23 percent in the last eight years.

Type 1 diabetes is an autoimmune disease often triggered by viruses. The virus causes the pancreas to no longer produce insulin, thus creating a dependency on outside sources for the hormone, typically provided through injections or a pump (type 1 also goes by the name insulin-dependent diabetes mellitus). Type 1 diabetes initially was only seen in children, which is why it was previously known as juvenile diabetes.

Type 2 diabetes is typically caused by age and poor lifestyle choices. The pancreas starts to show signs of wear and tear when it clocks too much overtime throughout the years. Medication and lifestyle changes are the preferred treatment methods for type 2 diabetes, which is also known as non-insulin dependent diabetes mellitus, since insulin is not required to manage the disease.

It is important to note that type 2 diabetics can also become insulin dependent if lifestyle changes are not made and/or the prescribed medications no longer prove effective. Type 2 diabetes was previously known as adult onset diabetes, because we mostly saw these cases in adults. Unfortunately, the terms juvenile and adult onset are no longer used, because more and more young people are getting type 2 diabetes from poor dietary choices and sedentary lifestyles.

With that information at hand, I was anxious to hear why type 1 diabetes was on the rise.

"Bugs."

"Superbugs?" I texted back.

"They're not saying that. Just weakened immune systems leading to more viruses."

It makes sense. Autoimmune disease requires an initiator and an activator. There are many people who live with a predisposition towards autoimmune disease all their life (eg. genetics), but if an activator never turns it on, they can live their lives free of the disease. Viruses and low vitamin D levels are just two examples of activators that top the list.

Now, I'm going to completely switch gears and tell you about a different study I also read around the same time that Erika and I had that conversation. It is no surprise to anyone that loneliness causes a decline in mental health, presenting symptoms such as stress, anxiety, and depression. Recently, studies suggest that loneliness is also affecting our physical health by causing greater inflammation and weakened immune systems. This leaves our bodies with a decreased ability to fight disease.[1]

Loneliness Sent You a Friend Request

There is a lot of good to Facebook. Since the social media outlet launched in 2004, people have been able to stay connected to loved ones, share pictures, and voice opinions on various topics. From personal experience, I have also known Facebook to be isolating. It sparks insecurity and jealousy from within.

"Why doesn't my family smile for family pictures (or at least look at the camera)?"

"Why doesn't my husband buy me expensive presents for my birthday?"

"Why don't we ever get to go on vacation to exotic islands?"

"Why doesn't my dinner look like the one my friend posted?"

"Why wasn't I invited to that party? All of those people are my friends too!"

"Why isn't my kid better at sports?"

"Why don't I look that way in a bikini?"

At times, I found that what was meant to create a feeling of connectedness actually lead to a sense of jealous competition, and I lost the contest every single time. I started to doubt the good in my own life, replacing gratitude with discontent. It was an ugly place.

Social media and texting have now become the dominant ways to communicate with others. Rarely do people pick up the phone to engage in an actual conversation anymore. When is the last time you had friends or family in your home? Is "company" even a word used in 2019? What about Sunday dinners? What about meals without phones? The saddest sight to see is a family (moms and dads included) looking at their phones instead of looking at each other.

Jim and I took the kids out to dinner a few years ago with the intention of spending quality time with the whole family. Needless to say, we were shocked when the waitress handed Jim and I menus and each kid a device to play on without even asking our permission first! We didn't go out to watch the tops of our kids' heads while they each played their own video game. Even though we were all present around the table, no one was having a conversation and it felt extremely lonely.

So, Facebook having an effect on the onset of diabetes isn't a far leap once you see my point of reference. Facebook can cause loneliness, which causes weakened immune systems, which allow for the growth of viruses, which are an activator for autoimmune disease. Type 1 diabetes is an autoimmune disease.

Our pastor recently showed us the image of Maslow's Hierarchy, a pictorial representation that reveals people's motivation levels to achieve specific needs. Our most basic, shown at the base of the triangle, is for physical survival and is what initially motivates our behaviors. Once that level is met, we can work on meeting our security needs. We cannot move up the scale until the needs of each section are met. For example, it's virtually impossible to improve our health if we aren't even sure how, or even if, we are going to be able to eat today.[2]

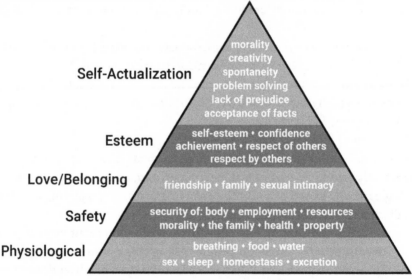

What I find fascinating about this graph is that the ego—otherwise known as self-esteem—cannot be met until community is achieved. If there is no connection within a community, self-confidence is at risk. Self-confidence is a crucial component for an individual to live his or her best life and it is what allows human beings to take risks and experience life to its fullest.

Loneliness absolutely has an affect on wellbeing. Do you feel lonely? Does social media actually cause more isolation than connectedness for you? Maybe it's time to ditch the screen and form real connectedness with those who are most important to you. We recently ran a 31-day health challenge at my practice to celebrate National Nutrition Month. In addition to challenging patients to eat more produce, increase water consumption, and meal plan, we also asked them to limit screen time and engage in more face-to-face conversations. Treating our bodies and each other well always leads to greater physical, mental, and emotional health. You get to make the choice to engage in more meaningful forms of communication. It's time to build your community and very possibly, lower your risk of developing diabetes.

eat

Sticky Situations

About six years ago, Jim and I were trying to decide where to go on our family vacation. The kids were young—my oldest six, and the twins not yet one—so we wanted to go somewhere fairly close and low key, but we also wanted to go to a place we had never visited before. We decided on Williamsburg, Virginia.

It took us forever to get there. No one really tells you about what travel with a large family will be like before you decide to have one. Parents of an odd number of kids face a specific challenge, also known as "the middle seat." This is where all the inter-sibling touching takes place.

Parents of two and four kids may not understand this challenge, because there is normally an open seat between the two window seats in the back row(s). This space allows for a touch-free zone between all children. Once you put a third child into the mix, forget about it. This is why parents with three kids gravitate toward a minivan. It's not because they particularly need the space, it's because they need their sanity.

Having five kids carries the same challenge. We would place both twins in the middle row captain chairs for easy transitions in and out of their car seats, but that meant the three boys were in the back ... together ... touching one another ... nonstop. You know what happens next—touching leads to yelling, yelling leads to fighting, and fighting leads to crying (both them and me).

So, after a six-hour car ride where everyone wound up exhausted, restless, and hungry, we arrived in Williamsburg. We decided to grab something to eat to restore everyone's moods and blood sugars. We found a restaurant called Red Hot & Blue. As it turned out, Red Hot & Blue was the perfect restaurant for our family since the prices were affordable and everyone could find something enjoyable on the menu.

The hostess offered us a booth if we wanted to be seated right away and we agreed without hesitation. We shuffled into a small booth—Parker and I on one side and Jim between Jake and Ben on the other side. The girls were each in their own highchairs at the end of the table.

The waitress brought out the children's menus along with some crayons to keep the boys happy. Our small booth quickly became inundated with art supplies, papers, drinks, plates, and silverware, but Jim and I tried to overlook the stress from the chaotic table and just relish in the fact that we had all made it there alive after being cooped up in a car for so long.

Just when we thought our table couldn't get any more crammed, our food came out and everyone started reaching around for condiments, silverware, and drinks. Jim has done an amazing job at introducing our kids to condiments, so the boys were grabbing every sticky barbecue sauce they could grab with their tiny hands. Jim kept telling them to sit still and wait for his help, but they were just too excited and hungry to wait.

In typical two-year-old fashion, Ben kept grabbing Jim's shirt to help himself sit into a position of feasting, Jim's blood boiling as he watched his shirt stain more and more with sticky barbecue sauce.

Right on cue, Charley had enough of her highchair and started crying. My family doesn't know how to do anything quietly. Not wanting Charley to amplify the noise coming from our corner of the restaurant, I quickly snatched her from the highchair in hopes of quieting her down.

Quick side note: I think babies have a sixth sense, knowing when their mamas are about to eat a hot meal. It doesn't matter if they are already fed and changed; if they see steam coming off of a plate we are about to eat, they shut that down so fast by screaming for attention.

It didn't take Bella long to realize that she was still stuck in her highchair, so she started wailing too. Jim looked at me as if to question what I was going to do about this situation, so I reminded him that I already had my baby, and that Bella was his responsibility. He tried to argue that he was taking care of Ben and was already a sticky mess, but Bella only began to cry louder. Defeated, he picked up Bella, overstuffing our booth of five with two infants. Thankfully, Jake was able to feed and entertain himself through the whole fiasco, as we tended to the other four children.

For just a few moments, there was peace among us. The girls quieted down enough for us to get in a few bites and we thought we were in the clear.

Once again, God had a sense of humor and decided He wasn't quite done with us yet. In one fell swoop, Ben reached across the table, grabbed the sticky barbecue sauce bottle and knocked Jim's full glass of lemonade over, the sticky fruit juice spilling down the table and onto Jim's lap.

His eyes widening, Jim grabbed any napkin he could find, but most of the napkins were wadded up into balls of barbecue. Meanwhile, Bella began to cry as the sticky liquid started to pour on her legs and I just lost it.

The more I laughed, the less I could control it, and the angrier Jim got, which just made me laugh even harder, starting the cycle all over again. There was nothing he could do but accept his fate and wait for the waitress to come over with more napkins, because he was wedged in a small booth sandwiched between three kids. I should have taken a picture of Jim when we left the restaurant, although thinking about it now, there was no way he would have let me permanently document that moment.

Clutter Creates Stress

This story illustrates the idea that clutter creates stress and ultimately impacts our experience. Since our dining adventure was an isolated event, we can laugh, but for many people, a messy eating area is an everyday reality.

What does your eating space look like? Is it clean or cluttered? The latter leads to chaos and chaos equals stress. Food and stress do not go well together. Think about the condition of your dining room table. Some people use it as a dumping ground for mail and papers. In our house, it is where the kids do homework and art projects. I'm constantly moving things off the table so we have room to eat, but there have been times I have been lazy and just moved things to the side. I always regret those times, because my mind gravitates to the mess and I soon find myself thinking about the chaos around the rest of the house.

I recently had the pleasure of meeting with one of my patients and explaining to him the benefits of getting away from eating his lunch at his desk and moving to a clean table without a computer screen monopolizing both physical space on the desk and mental space in his brain. My patient explained it was common in his work culture for everyone to eat at their desks for lunch and that he usually caught up with Yahoo! or Facebook during his break.

He agreed to move his lunch destination to see if he noticed anything different about his meal experience and to report back with his findings. The following week, he walked into my office giddy with excitement to tell me his story.

"I thought a lot about what you said, so I decided to try eating my lunch away from my desk," he said. "I invited a coworker I have known for years to join me, telling him my nutritionist is making me eat lunch away from my desk and asked if he wanted to come. He agreed and we found an empty conference room."

"Let me tell you Adrianne, it was one of the nicest lunches I've had in a really long time. I have known this guy for six years, but I learned more about him in those 30 minutes by having a face-to-face conversation than I have in years of seeing him around the office. We both enjoyed our lunch so much that we invited another guy to join us the following day and the same thing happened again! I not only enjoyed my lunch so much more, but the conversations we had were great. A couple of us at work decided we're going to do lunch this way more often."

I was so excited for him! Just a small adjustment like getting up and eating lunch away from his desk had a profound impact on his day and relationships.

I challenge you to do the same. Ignore the work culture of eating at your desk and create your own space to recharge and cultivate meaningful relationships. I guarantee you will come back refreshed and rejuvenated, finding greater satisfaction in both your vocation and your relationships with others.

repeat

Simplify Your Environment

Think about the last time you went to the movie theater and ordered popcorn (or any food for that matter). As the movie previews start, you begin enjoying the hot, buttery flavor. Roughly a quarter into the movie, you reach into the bag to eat more popcorn only to realize it's all gone. You temporarily panic and think, "I need more popcorn," despite having consumed the entire bag. Why? Because you don't remember eating the popcorn and if your brain misses out on an experience, it wants a do-over.

I ask my patients how the 16th bite of their bag of snack tasted during a movie or TV show. Every time, without fail, I get a blank stare in response. The answer, of course, is that the patient doesn't know, because he or she wasn't paying attention, because of the distraction caused by the movie.

You have heard of distracted driving, but I need to introduce you to distracted eating. This violation is defined as engaging in an activity while eating food, leading the eater to not be fully present and aware of how much he or

116

she is consuming.

In my experience, screens are the most common culprit of distracted eating—TV screens, computer screens, and phone screens. They each provide a level of distraction or escape that takes our attention off of what we are eating, leading us to overconsumption.

Enter the third S of mindful eating: **simplify your environment**.

What distractions do you need to eliminate so that you can be fully present with your meal? Do you catch up on emails and current events during your lunch break? Do you scroll through social media at night while eating a bowl of ice cream? If so, you are missing out on experiencing the full pleasure of your meal and the opportunity to be in tune with the signals your body will give you when you approach fullness.

Television is perhaps the most dangerous activity in which to indulge when it comes to our health.

First, it's an activity that many people engage in on a daily basis, often for multiple hours at a time, leading to a sedentary lifestyle.

Second, there are so many commercials selling us on the idea that we need advertised foods to validate our days or worthiness. Advertisements prey on our emotions and fatigue with images of high-calorie items promising happiness and love. Think about it; have you ever seen a real-life hamburger from McDonald's look like the one in the commercial? Have you ever finished a fast food hamburger and felt like frolicking in a field of flowers all while smiling and laughing with your loved ones?

Next time you watch TV at night, count how many commercials you see for eating fruits and vegetables. I once heard the advice, "If there's a commercial for it, don't eat it."

Perhaps the most dangerous part about eating in front of the TV is the association it creates. If you are in the habit of eating dinner in front of the TV, as many of my patients are, your brain will start to create associations, pairing the two activities together. This becomes challenging when you are watching TV at a time other than a meal, because your brain notices something is missing and will prompt you to question why you are not eating. You may go to the kitchen to grab something even in the *absence* of hunger. This could be why some people feel bored when they are watching TV and seek out food. Not only have they just watched 20 commercials about food, but they subconsciously notice their hands aren't doing anything purposeful. Here comes eating to the rescue—providing us with something to do.

As noted previously, I have a fair share of patients who do not take lunch breaks, eating at their desks in front of computer screens, instead of going to the break room, or somewhere else more peaceful. This scenario is no different than eating in front of the TV. It is a common misconception that working through lunch will lead to higher productivity, but studies show the opposite to be the case. Fewer than 20 percent of American workers regularly step away for a midday meal, and 39 percent usually eat at their desks, according to a survey done by Right Management.[3] Moving away from your desk creates a mental break your mind needs. That break results in increased creativity, improved concentration, and the ability to maintain a longer attention span. All of these positive outcomes lead to decreased stress, fatigue, and burnout.

Feeling overwhelmed and stressed can lead to increased visits to the break room for snacks. Since the food provided in most company break rooms is of the vending machine variety or a collection of all the items people don't want in their house, the story never ends well. Take advantage of your company's lunchroom or outdoor picnic area for a much-needed mental break.

How can you simplify your environment right now? Is it creating a clean, dining table space? Is it eating your lunch in the break room? Is it eating your dinner at the table with the TV turned off? Start with one area and observe how remaining present with your meal affects your satisfaction with the taste and quantity of your food.

choose your plan

Affirmation

Repeat this statement every day this week:

*"I will consciously work to declutter my mind
and my environment when I eat."*

Action

If you work outside of the home, eat lunch away from your desk this week. For every meal you eat in your home, make the effort to clean off the table before enjoying your meal.

Achieve

Take a break from social media this week. Bonus points if you initiate conversations through actual phone calls rather than text messages.

Analyze

Find a way to simplify your environment this week by avoiding combining screen time with meal or snack time. Journal about the changes you are feeling in your mind and body surrounding the switch from your normal routine.

Accountability

Answer the below questions in your dedicated healthy lifestyle journal:

What change did you attempt to make this week?

Were you happy with the results?

What challenges did you encounter?

How would you do things differently next time?

5-star recipes
Creamy Tomato Soup

When I think of comfort foods with my family around the table, I think of foods I ate growing up. The combination of grilled cheese and tomato soup was one of my favorites as a kid. This twist on a classic gets its rich, creamy flavors from beans, but no one will ever know unless they see you make it. Say goodbye to condensed soup from a can! Since this is thicker in consistency, it can also stand in as a tomato sauce or pizza sauce in a pinch.

Makes 8 servings

Ingredients

2–3 TBS olive oil
1 large yellow onion, chopped
3 large carrots, peeled and chopped
¼ tsp crushed red pepper flakes
2 cloves garlic, minced
2 tsp dried basil
2 TBS tomato paste
3 (28 oz.) cans whole tomatoes, with liquid
½–1 cup chopped roasted red peppers, drained
4 cups vegetable broth
1 cup canned Great Northern or cannellini beans, rinsed and drained
1 TBS unsalted butter
1 TBS brown sugar
Salt and pepper, to taste
10–15 roughly chopped, fresh basil leaves

Directions

1. In a Dutch oven or soup pot, warm the olive oil over medium heat. Add the onion, carrots, and red pepper flakes and cook, stirring occasionally, until the vegetables are tender, about 8 to 10 minutes.
2. Add the garlic and dried basil; cook for an additional minute.
3. Add the tomato paste, tomatoes, roasted peppers, and vegetable broth and stir to combine. Increase the heat to medium-high and bring the mixture to a simmer. Cook for 25 minutes, reducing the heat as necessary to

maintain a gentle simmer and stirring occasionally.

4. Remove the pot from the heat and let it cool for a few minutes. Carefully transfer the mixture to a blender.
5. Add the beans, butter, sugar, salt, and black pepper to the blender. Blend the soup until smooth.
6. Taste soup and adjust seasonings as needed. Add basil, blend once more and serve.

Source: Adapted from Taste of Home[4]

White Bean Salad

Packing lunch everyday—the physical act of packing and the mental stamina it takes to come up with an idea—is daunting, so bean salads are my quick go-to solution. I typically triple the recipe on Sundays so we can dip out of them all week. This recipe is so easy to make and you can mix up the veggies and cheese for some variety.

Makes 2 servings

Ingredients

2 TBS olive oil
1 TBS lemon juice
Salt and pepper, to taste
½ onion, diced
Fresh parsley, chopped
1 (15 oz.) can cannelloni beans, rinsed and drained
Grape tomatoes, halved
Cucumber, quartered
Feta cheese (optional)

Directions

1. Mix the first five ingredients in a small bowl. Allow the flavors to marry while chopping the vegetables.
2. Add the remaining ingredients to a large bowl.
3. Pour the marinade from Step 1 over the bean mixture from Step 2 and toss to serve.

Source: Adapted from SimplyRecipes.com[5]

lesson 10

Mind Your Taste Buds

"Show up in every single moment like you're meant to be there."
—*Marie Forleo*

The above quote screams confidence, which is why I gravitate toward it so much. I have a decent amount of self-confidence, but when doubt starts to creep into my mental space, I become mush. People who can walk into a room and command it fascinate me. I am in awe of people who know what they want and then aggressively go after it.

Whether it's with business, life, or food, having intentionality exudes confidence and leadership. A professional athlete doesn't step onto the field "hoping" to do well; he commands it by being intentional with his skill and routine. If we want to have the confidence to execute, we have to trust the work that we put into our practice will yield the desired results.

When it comes to food, we have to trust that our body knows what it's doing. We have to let the distractions of our minds and other people take a backseat so we can be present in the moment. Making deliberate and conscious choices both before the meal and between bites allows us to command the mealtime.

Commanding a meal is not meant to be an aggressive action, but rather, it opens the gate to freedom and enjoyment. Many conventional diets take the joy out of eating, replacing it with a list of do's and don'ts. It's time we bring a little fun back to the party and appreciate the flavors and joy that food has to offer.

nourish

Savor Your Food

It's time for the main event. The fourth S of our mindful eating journey is **savor**. I frequently go over these powerful lessons of the mind with my patients. When I got to "savor," I had a patient stop me once, mid-sentence.

"No need to discuss this one," he gushed. "When I eat, I am totally into it. I'm all in. I will close my eyes even if I'm at a restaurant just so I can enjoy every ounce of flavor."

He even went as far as physically demonstrating how he sat, eyes closed, with a huge smile across his face. He was so funny!

Isn't this how it should be? Whenever I tell this story, I always feel so invigorated, imagining him enjoying the moment by simply tasting his food.

Can you say you share the same experience? I know I can't. Looking back, when I threw the whole pack of M&Ms into my mouth all at once, I can honestly say I did not enjoy a single piece of it. I was too busy trying to pretend I wasn't eating.

There are also the occasions when I eat food just because it's present. The food may not even be tasty, but I eat it anyway, just for the simple reason that it's in front of me. Everyone has his or her own opinion on the better option: a hard or soft chocolate chip cookie. I prefer soft. How many times have I been to a party or event where they served hard cookies and I ate them anyway? If I had taken my patient's approach of closing my eyes and tasting every bite—chances are I would have realized I wasn't enjoying the food. This bears the question: if you're not enjoying the food, why are you eating it?

My recommendation to patients is to only eat homemade food items at parties. Why? Because they usually taste better. People have good intentions about making food, but most are pressed for time and end up buying something at the store. You can purchase store-made items any day of the year. They are not special.

I also have found that if I don't enjoy the food I'm eating I will want to repeat the behavior with hopes of creating a different outcome. Eating mediocre foods never ends well. For example, we went to a benefit one night to support a local charity. After the meal, there was an assortment of bite-size desserts available, but none that particularly interested me (it was all cream puffs and I'm more of a brownie or pie kind of girl). I grabbed one of them just to eat something sweet, but didn't enjoy it. After the silent auction, I

124

asked Jim if we could go out for ice cream. He looked at me and asked if I was kidding, reminding me of the piece of dessert I had just consumed. I told him I wanted a do-over. When we don't enjoy the experience we are more likely to continue eating until we reach the desired amount of pleasure.

To clarify, reaching a state of pleasure is not a bad thing! We are wired to seek pleasure and food can be an opportunity to acquire that satisfaction. Most people who come into my office tell me they love food so much that it is the reason why they are overweight. If I ask them to rank how much pleasure they derive from eating on a scale of 1 to 10, most will give it an 11 or higher.

Although I tell this group of patients that it's important to enjoy their food, we do need to find a way to knock it down a few notches. I find it interesting to analyze eating habits when it comes to seeking pleasure. Most of us don't realize our habits may be outside the norm, because we have been "in the habit" of doing them for so long.

I have my own eating quirks that I wasn't aware of until recently. We were at a buffet for an event and I put a variety of foods onto my plate. I was particularly excited about the chicken piccata since it is one of my favorite dishes, and the mashed potatoes looked delicious as well. The buffet contained green beans and pasta which also went onto my plate.

One habit I developed during my childhood was to eat one food at a time before moving on to the next item. I eat my food in the order of least to most favorite so I can save the best item for last. I never questioned my eating style, because no one challenged it.

That particular day, when I was trying to be more mindful about my meals, I was enlightened. I started with the pasta first, because it visually wasn't my favorite thing on the plate. Next, I moved to the huge pile of green beans (I love my veggies, which is why I took a lot of them, but compared to mashed potatoes and chicken piccata, it won third place). As I moved to the mashed potatoes, I started to notice I was beginning to feel a little full.

Oh no! I started to panic, because I told myself before the meal I was going to stop eating when I got the signal of fullness. However, mentally I was not ready to stop eating, because I was still enjoying the mashed potatoes. Plus, I hadn't even gotten to my favorite yet—the chicken picatta.

Clearly, this method of saving the best for last was no longer going to work for me, because if I get full before my plate is clear, I will always miss out on my favorite part or most likely eat past fullness. I did what any other person would do (or at least I like to tell myself that); I took one more bite of mashed potatoes and a couple bites of the chicken, because I wanted to taste it. Yes, I ate past fullness, but I learned a valuable lesson in the process.

This story reminds me of a patient I once consulted. He shared the same frustration of eating past fullness when it came to tasty meals. He asked me, "I'm finding it really hard to stop eating when my stomach gives me fullness signals, but my tongue says it's not done tasting yet."

I knew exactly what he meant! He continued, "But, I think I figured it out. When my stomach gives me the fullness signal, I tell myself I can have three more bites. It's a compromise between ignoring the signal completely and honoring my body's cues."

I was so proud of him for coming up with that genius approach. Think about it ... the same works for kids when you are leaving a destination. If you tell a child who is having fun, "It's time to go now," you will always be met with whining and resistance. "Oh, come on, just five more minutes! I'm not done playing yet."

However, if you give the child a warning and tell him, "Johnny, in 10 minutes, we're going to be leaving. Finish up what you're doing and start putting the toys away," he has time to mentally prepare for playtime to end.

It's the same with food. When you try to shut down a fun time in your mouth, your brain will always meet you with some resistance. However, give it a warning sign and you're more likely to come to terms with the party ending.

A Few Questions to Ponder

One of the best pieces of advice I heard about savoring foods is to remember that your taste buds are on your tongue, not in your stomach. We have a variety of taste buds to help us detect and enjoy the flavors of food. Use them! Let your food spend more time in your mouth than in your stomach. Close your eyes so you can really taste each bite you take.

When you're sitting down to a meal, Dr. Susan Albers reminds us to ask ourselves four very important questions:

1. Do I like the way this looks?
2. Do I like the way this smells?
3. Do I like the way it tastes?
4. Do I like the consistency?

If the food is not bringing you joy, move on. If you decide to save the best for last, make sure your portions are small so you get to the finish line. If you are met with a fullness signal and mentally aren't ready to finish, try giving your taste buds two or three last compromising bites and see how it changes your experience.

eat

Singles vs. Homeruns

Patients frequently ask me, "Can you give me a healthy dessert recipe?" This lights me up right away, because I know the answer. However, much to my disappointment, the patient usually interjects, reading my mind, "Oh, but not fruit; something else."

I typically reply in frustration, "But, that's the healthiest dessert!"

Of course, my patients don't mean any harm with the added disclaimer, but it speaks truth to what kind of foods our society has grown to covet. Just recently, I did a grocery store tour with a patient and while we were in the cereal aisle, he commented that his kids would never eat the types of cereal I select for my children.

I replied, "That's because your kids are used to homeruns."

Let me explain this concept more using the following example. When you eat fresh strawberries from the garden, there is a certain nuance to each bite. Some berries are extra sweet, while others are a bit on the bland side. Some have a warm center and are the perfect balance between firm and soft, while others are a little riper and mushy. Each bite is a surprise as you anticipate the flavor and consistency you're going to taste next. The berry is appropriately sweet and satisfying. It's like hitting a single in the game of baseball. A single is both acceptable and celebrated by the fans. My dad, who was also my softball coach, always told us that while homeruns are great, singles are what win games.

Now, let's switch gears and talk about Dairy Queen strawberry sundaes. We all know you are not getting fresh strawberries from the garden on top of your vanilla ice cream, but instead, a processed, lab-created sugar berry. Each gram of sugar excites and ignites pleasure centers in your brain. You can go to any Dairy Queen in the nation with an expectation of flavor and it will be met every single time. You don't have to worry that the topping will be less than satisfying, because it is manufactured in a processing plant that can guarantee consistency with each bite. Because it is a manmade product and has chemicals and processed sugars to attack pleasure centers of your brain, it's like eating a homerun every time. Homeruns are exciting and thrilling for fans in the sport of baseball. Nothing brings the crowd to their feet like an out-of-the-park home run.

The problem with the majority of foods we eat on a day-to-day basis is they are prepackaged homeruns. When given the option to eat a God-made food from nature, we tend to look the other way, and instead gravitate toward those foods that provide the most reward. We are no longer satisfied with singles; we want a homerun every time.

In the case of my patient's kids in the grocery store, they were so used to eating sugary cereals that offering them one with less sugar would be a letdown.

When I first started working as a dietitian, I partnered with two other business owners in the area to create a nutrition weight loss program. We developed a 12-week program, focusing on weight loss methods that would provide quick results. For the first two weeks of the program, we restricted all forms of carbohydrates with the exception of vegetables. It was grueling for our participants to get rid of all the junk, but a good kick-start for most of them to say goodbye to processed foods. On the third week of the program, we introduced berries as a way to acclimate them back into a healthy, all-encompassing diet. You should have heard the comments…

"These are the best strawberries I have ever tasted in my life!"

"I have never in my life had a raspberry so sweet before. Did they always taste this way?"

"Why have I never noticed how sweet blueberries were before?"

I would secretly chuckle at these comments, knowing all along the reason the clients were responding in that way was because they had new perspectives. When you take all the junk out of your diet, then berries can stand to be what they were created to be … a sweet treat! No need for chocolate when you have a nice, sweet berry at your fingertips.

The problem is processed sugary treats will always make berries pale in comparison. Take the treats out of the equation and the berries become enough. The only way to make singles be enough is to stop eating homeruns so frequently.

Now, this isn't to say you can never eat a homerun for the rest of your life. That's absurd. Homeruns should be a once-in-a-while treat. What fun would the baseball game be if every single batter hit a homerun? Maybe it would be fun at first, but over time it would lose its excitement. Eating processed foods all the time may also appear fun at first. But over time, you'll notice you're a lot more sluggish and have an expanding waistline.

When my patient asked me how I get my kids to eat the cereals with less sugar, the answer was quite simple. They don't have another option. If given the choice between Cheerios and Fruit Loops, my kids would always pick Fruit Loops. However, since that is not one of the options, the Cheerios work just fine.

I challenge you to look at your own pantry and fridge for homeruns. These are processed foods that are high in sugar, salt, and fat. If you find yourself gravitating toward these items more than healthier alternatives—such as fruits and vegetables, which can also provide sweetness, crunch, and texture—then maybe it's time to evaluate what foods you are bringing into the house on a regular basis.

Remember, singles win games.

repeat

Small Portions, High Prices

My friend's husband is a chef. I'm not talking just any old chef. I mean, he's a grandmaster in the kitchen.

When he first started culinary school, my family and I were his guinea pigs, and let me tell you, his natural abilities blew us all away. His talent has taken him to Nantucket, the Hamptons, and our nation's capital, and I'm proud to say he's now opening up his own restaurant.

Needless to say, he knows the industry. One night, our conversation led us to the topic of expensive restaurants.

"Do you ever wonder why the portions appear to be smaller the more expensive the restaurant?" he asked.

"Well, I guess I never really thought about it," I admitted, "I always just chalked it up to the simple reason, 'Because they can.'"

He proceeded to explain.

There have been studies created to assess when an individual reaches his or her peak level of enjoyment based on how many bites of a food he or she has taken.[1]

Let's use an example with a plate of ravioli. Based on a "pleasure scale" of 1 to 10 (1 being the lowest amount of pleasure and 10 being the highest), you rate your first bite as a 9, because you're still gathering information about the item. Maybe it has a hint of sweetness in the filling or a flash of spice in the sauce that you only notice at the end of your chewing experience.

You enjoyed your bite, but it was more of an information-gathering bite. You realize you like what you tasted. You go in for the second bite and this time it is a clear 10. You know what to expect. You may have even started salivating before you got your fork to your mouth. You instinctually react in one of two ways: tell your dinner partner that he or she simply must try what you are eating, because it is the best ravioli you ever had in your entire life and you want to share the experience; or, tell your dinner partner to not even think about taking a bite of your food or you'll rip his or her head off! This plate is all yours.

Bite number 3 is also rated a 10, because it is just that amazing. Bite number 4 could be a 10, but it could also be a 9. Now, it doesn't mean you're not enjoying what you are eating; it's just that you are no longer at the peak of your experience. With each successive bite, your enjoyment of the food will continue to decline.

This scenario is likely familiar to many, especially when thinking about a buffet. By the time you are on your fourth plate, you are no longer hungry. You are also no longer enjoying what you are eating. You are simply trying to get your money's worth. You may leave the buffet feeling stuffed, sick, or even have the need to unbutton your pants. It's not your finest moment, and all you can think about is taking a nap. You leave the buffet telling yourself, "I don't ever want to do that again. I'm never overeating like this ever again." Yet, once enough time goes by, you forget (sort of like the childbirth experience; am I right ladies?).

With a fine-dining establishment, you are only given enough bites to stay at the peak of your experience. You leave the restaurant groaning, "If I could have only had two more bites of those raviolis … they were amazing … we have to tell Andrew and Danielle to try this place—they would love it … I can't wait to come here again!"

This experience is very different from the buffet, where you swear off all food. When you leave a buffet, your first thought isn't to tell everyone you know about the restaurant; it's how to recline the back of the car seat low enough to get comfortable.

When you only have small volumes of food, you are also less likely to gobble it. I have yet to see someone with a plate of four raviolis consume all four pieces of pasta in one bite. That's absurd. When only given four raviolis, we typically try to extend the experience by cutting them into quarters. We slow down our pace—we may even close our eyes—and move the food around our mouths as to extract every ounce of flavor the food provides. We are more in tune with the flavors of the dish, leading to a higher pleasure value for the entire dining experience. We usually leave feeling comfortable, not stuffed.

This past summer, Jim and I visited a tapas-style restaurant. Since neither of us had dined at this type of restaurant before, we asked the waitress for help. The waitress explained we should order one dish at a time—since each dish was meant to be shared—and after we split the dish, we could order another item to try.

That meal format was highly appealing to us, as we had a babysitter and no set time to return home. We ordered our first plate—roasted Brussels sprouts—and waited for our food while drinking a glass of wine and enjoying each other's company. The outdoor seating was quaint and entertaining, complimenting the serene weather favorably.

When the waitress arrived with a saucer (not salad plate) of sprouts, Jim and I looked at each other as if to say, "That's it?" Nevertheless, we proceeded to divide the plate in two.

We took our time eating the delicious veggies and enjoyed the ambiance. The evening was turning out to be more fun than we expected! Our waitress returned about 10 minutes later, and asked if we were ready to order our next plate. This time we chose seafood jambalaya and the flavors did not disappoint. Because our portions were small, every bite was a 10! We shared two more plates throughout the evening and left the restaurant comfortably satiated. Much like our bites, we rated our overall experience a 10, wanting to tell everyone about our memorable evening.

Next time you eat a meal, think about approaching it in a more intentional way. Take note of the amount of pleasure you receive from each bite. When your body tells you that you are no longer receiving pleasure, move on or stop. The results might fascinate you and change your eating behaviors.

choose your plan

Affirmation

Repeat this statement every day this week:

"Singles win games."

Action

At your next meal, make a conscious effort to utilize all of your taste buds. Move the food around your mouth and intentionally taste each bite. If the food isn't bringing you pleasure, move on.

Achieve

This week, remove all "homerun" desserts and replace them with fresh fruit.

Analyze

Choose a meal this week and rate each bite on your own pleasure scale. Identify at which point your satisfaction with different foods begins to wane. Notice how your stomach's fullness impacts your perceived pleasure. Write your findings in your journal.

Accountability

Answer the below questions in your dedicated healthy lifestyle journal:

What change did you attempt to make this week?

Were you happy with the results?

What challenges did you encounter?

How would you do things differently next time?

5-star recipes

Brussels Sprouts and Butternut Squash with Bacon

Yes, bacon is an ingredient in one of my healthy recipes (it's okay when used in small amounts)! Because there isn't a ton of bacon, you end up savoring each bite. One of my patients shared this recipe during a session, claiming her boys loved it. Turns out my kids were fans too! Why wouldn't they be? Everyone loves bacon! This dish is a perfect side dish for a busy night or on your Thanksgiving table.

Makes 4 servings

Ingredients

1 lb. Brussels sprouts, halved

1 lb. butternut squash, cubed

3 slices uncooked bacon, diced

Directions

1. Place Brussels sprouts and butternut squash on sheet pan.

2. Arrange bacon on top of vegetables

3. Bake at 400°F for 35 minutes, turning over with spatula halfway through baking. Veggies should be fork tender when finished cooking.

Chicken Piccata

As I mentioned in the beginning of this section, chicken piccata is one of my favorite dishes. This variation is quick to pull together without sacrificing flavor.

Makes 4 servings

Ingredients

1 lb. thin sliced chicken breast

3 TBS flour

¼ tsp salt

¼ tsp pepper

2 TBS olive oil

6 garlic cloves, minced

½ cup white wine (alternatively use chicken broth)

¼ cup low-sodium chicken broth

2 (10 oz.) bags spinach

1 TBS unsalted butter

Juice of 1 lemon

4 tsp capers, rinsed and drained

2 TBS fresh parsley, chopped

Directions

1. Combine flour with salt and pepper in a shallow dish. Coat chicken in the flour mixture.

2. In medium skillet, heat 1 tsp oil over medium-high heat and add chicken. Cook until browned on both sides, approximately 7 to 10 minutes. Remove chicken from pan and cover with foil to keep warm until later.

3. Add 2 of the minced garlic cloves to empty skillet and stir for 20 seconds. Add wine (or broth); cook for three minutes. Add chicken broth; cook for 2 minutes.

4. In large skillet add remaining oil and minced garlic. Sauté for 1 minute over medium heat until fragrant. Add spinach in batches tossing with kitchen tongs until wilted. When finished cooking, turn heat to low to keep warm.

5. Remove skillet with the sauce in it from the heat. Stir in butter, lemon juice, capers, and parsley. Divide sautéed spinach between four plates and place chicken breast on top. Spoon sauce over chicken. Serve with additional lemon wedges if desired.

lesson 11

Choosing Happiness

"Only I can change my life. No one can do it for me."
—Carol Burnett

I may not be able to choose the circumstances in my life, but I will always be able to choose how I react to them. It's such a wise concept, but so incredibly hard to execute. Some circumstances are painful! As a result, I want to scream, cry, and eat my face off, because food has always temporarily made me feel better in times of sadness, anxiety, fear, or boredom.

I'm not exactly sure when I learned this was an acceptable coping mechanism. My parents were more likely to use food as a reward, taking us out for ice cream if we won a softball game rather than using it as a comfort tool. Yet, here I stand.

Changing this part of my life took a **long time**. It doesn't matter how conscious you are, how much awareness you have, or how much you read. This concept takes practice and more practice. Then, just when you think you've got it, you better get back out there and go practice again. It may take months or even years to rewrite your reaction, which takes a lot of patience (one of my most terrible weaknesses). You must learn to take the pain of a situation and use it for good instead of stuffing it down where no one can see, only to have it resurface at the most inconvenient moments. This choice is conscious and intentional. It means purposely choosing the hard road, knowing there will be healing on the other side.

Remember, good things can also come from pain. We learn empathy and compassion, which in turn, develops kindness. I can't wait until you see the power of kindness in this next section.

nourish

Sitting in the Suckiness

Three weeks after making the decision to compile these stories into a book, I lost one of my most favorite patients ever. After admitting herself into the hospital with shortness of breath, which they assumed was the beginning of a heart attack, she underwent various tests to rule out a cardiac diagnosis.

A PET scan revealed tumors lined all up and down both lungs. The cancer spread into her liver and her official diagnosis was Stage 4 esophageal cancer.

She texted me her diagnosis on October 4. On October 10, she was moved to hospice. On October 13, she met Jesus.

I didn't get to see her in the hospital. Her last form of communication with me was on October 7 via text. I lost a patient, but more importantly, I lost a friend, trusted confidant, and mentor. The immense grief I felt over the weeks following was overwhelming.

In the middle of all that, I lost my church home due to circumstances beyond my control. My church family for 17 years was no longer my family. We started visiting other churches, and every week, my family begged me to go back to our previous home church. Two months later, we were still trying to find a new home.

I felt like I was alone, carrying the burden of figuring everything out and not screwing up my kids in the process. On top of feeling isolated, I felt confused, betrayed, and an immense sadness, while I grieved for the two losses. The crushing grief from both losing a church home and family friend felt suffocating.

One night, I met with a client who shared her feelings of poor body image and how it impacted her life. Typically, I have a strict policy: "If you cry, I cry," and I have been known to share a tissue box with my patients. That particular night, as tears rolled down her cheeks, I felt absolutely nothing. I felt dead inside as I watched her cry and could not share in her sadness. It scared me. I didn't recognize myself. Was I becoming depressed? Was I becoming cold-hearted? I hated the feeling of not knowing the answers.

I have been fortunate to come across a lot of wisdom in my journey as a clinician. One quote came from a "Humans of New York" Facebook post:

"'If you could give one piece of advice to a large group of people, what would it be?'

136

"'Try your best to deal with life without medicating yourself.'

"'You mean drugs?'

"'I mean drugs, food, shopping, money, whatever. I ain't judging anybody, either. I was hooked on heroin for years. But now I've learned that every feeling will pass if you give it time. And if you learn to deal with your feelings, they'll pass by faster each time. So don't rush to cover them up, or you're never gonna learn.'"[1]

I came across this post five years ago, but it resonated with me, so I tucked away that wisdom for a future time. Now was the time. I decided to sit in the suckiness of my own feelings. I allowed myself to grieve, to feel pain, and to feel sadness. And you know what? It sucked just as much as you would expect. I cried a lot. I yelled a lot. I prayed a lot. I would find myself standing in the kitchen and then remind myself there was nothing food could do to change my feelings. So I would move to the sofa or outside on the back deck and just sit in the suckiness again, hoping the feelings would go away.

I relate the idea of waiting with my experience in the NICU. Four out of five kids spent time there after birth, and as much as I wanted to will my babies to get better, the only thing that actually worked was time. I would get so angry watching babies arrive to the NICU after my children and leave before us. It didn't seem fair.

I didn't want other babies to be sick for as long as my children were, but I was so scared and hurt that jealousy was my default emotion. No amount of whining, crying, or complaining was going to change the outcome. I just had to take it. It felt like getting beat up, but instead of swinging back, I just had to take the blows.

Over the next few weeks it was interesting to see how "dealing with my feelings" played out. All of that sitting and feeling led to a powerful realization: "The one thing good about all of this junk in my life is that this is the first time in 39 years I didn't eat through my feelings," I revealed to my friend, Carrie, over the phone about two weeks after implementing my new approach.

I have never been able to say that in my life. Most memorably, when I received the news my cousin had brain cancer, I found a huge spread of food on the counter with no recollection of taking it out of the fridge or how much I consumed.

Not eating my feelings in this latest case was a **huge** victory. It proved to me it could be done. It proved to me that I could move on. It gave me hope.

I shared this exact story with another patient who was struggling with a

137

binge-eating episode. As we were figuring out ways to bring her true feelings to the surface, rather than stuffing them away with food, I felt like I needed to be vulnerable and share my own struggles. She thanked me for telling her the story and after we wiped away our tears, we moved on to finding constructive solutions.

As I grabbed a tissue, I secretly welcomed myself back into the person I was prior to the month of suckiness. I would like to think that a few-week sabbatical outside of my comfort zone was better than a few months of pretending the feelings didn't exist only to have them resurface again and again.

I have always felt like I needed to have all the answers, especially in my field of work. After all, people are paying me to tell them what to do. I'm finding that when I change my job description from expert know-it-all to honest, vulnerable, partner consultant, the results are further reaching and longer lasting.

My choice to be vulnerable and allow someone else to see my pain was ultimately what allowed my client to open up and share hers. Once we were honest with each other, it created an opportunity for growth and healing. Too often, I think we're so concerned with presenting our best selves (remember those representatives from Lesson 4?) that we forget to present the self with which others can relate and find safety.

It's okay to not have your act together all the time. It's okay to feel sad in situations. That's why we live in community with one another—we are here to help each other. Our egos protect us from seeing and recognizing our true selves, because it can cause pain, disconnect, and confusion. Instead of telling yourself you're fine, it's okay to admit and acknowledge to yourself that you're not. Sit in the discomfort, not to add to the pain, but to move through the pain. When trouble finds you, I invite you to sit in your suckiness and see the difference it makes toward healing. You may find the feelings do pass by faster, just like that gentleman on Facebook said years ago.

eat

Smile

The fifth and final mindful eating method is to **smile**! I know what you're thinking ... there is always a cheesy tip in these acronym-based tools (or at least that's what I thought when I first heard it). Dr. Albers recommends smiling in between each bite as an additional method for slowing down. It totally makes sense if you think about it. I'm not going to take huge bites if I have to smile in between each forkful. I'm also going to chew more thoroughly to make sure I'm not flashing the bite of broccoli I just put in my mouth to everyone seated around me at the dinner table.

Taking smaller bites and chewing more thoroughly accomplishes the goals of staying present and being able to recognize the body's cues for fullness.

Smiling in between bites may appear kind of creepy to the people you're dining with. Instead, I'm going to take "smile" in a different direction. Remember when we talked about slowing down? One of the powerful and effective tools we added to our arsenals was to take a few deep, cleansing breaths before your meal to de-stress and set the tone for your pace. I'm going to add one additional step.

After you take your breaths, I want you to ask yourself, "Do I feel like smiling?" This is not the cheesy, "Here you go, Adrianne, are you happy now?" smile; it is a legitimate, "I feel good about what I'm about to do" smile.

For example, when I sit down to eat my avocado toast in the morning with a fried egg on top and a piece or two of fruit, I can smile knowing that my meal is nutritious, fulfilling, and tasty. However, there are also times when I'm feeling overwhelmed or stressed and grab a handful of tortilla chips. If I'm being honest, smiling doesn't feel authentic in those moments. It feels forced. If you're not in a good place emotionally and are not able to smile, I question if eating is the right activity for you in that moment.

A lot of times we eat for reasons other than hunger. We all do it and you are not a bad person for using food as a coping mechanism from time to time. The problem is, when we abuse it and use food as a coping mechanism **all the time** in every situation. Occasionally, we want to check out from our reality, and food can provide a numbing sensation that allows us to temporarily escape. It's a distraction.

Remember when you fell down and skinned your knee as a child? Your mom maybe gave you a cookie to make you stop crying. A hug would have worked here too, but the cookie distracted you and most likely quieted you down the fastest. I'm guilty for doing this to my own kids and had to make a conscious effort to find creative ways to soothe them that didn't involve food so as not to create an unhealthy association.

In my example of shoving M&M's in my mouth, I told you there were violations all over the place of mindful eating:

1. I was standing up to eat the candy.
2. I shoved the whole pack in my mouth all at once (there was nothing slow about the action).
3. I was hiding from my kids, creating a stressful eating environment.

4. I didn't enjoy one piece of that candy, because I was trying to hide the fact that it was in my mouth, and because I didn't enjoy it, I went back for more to repeat the experience.
5. The reason I ate the candy in the first place was because I was stressed out.

You see, I wasn't hungry. I was overwhelmed. Had I sat down, taken a few breaths and asked myself to smile, I would have had an opportunity to realize food wasn't the solution. Going outside for a walk, listening to some music, or even calling one of my friends would have been a much better antidote for my stress.

Eating as a Coping Mechanism

There are so many lists and ideas out there containing different things to do when you're stressed out. We keep returning to these lists, hoping to find a new idea we haven't tried. There are two problems with this strategy: we are trying to remember to use these alternative activities in a stressful moment, and we are not addressing the root cause of the problem itself.

I always tell patients, "If I was thinking clearly, I wouldn't need the coping mechanism." If we correctly identify the emotion—stress, anxiety, and/or boredom—we can create solutions that are appropriate and effective.

Human beings hate feeling uncomfortable. We rush to cover it up. What if we forced ourselves to sit in an uncomfortable state? What if we taught our kids, or our friends, to use language such as, "Hey, this situation sucks, I don't like the way this is making you feel and I wish it wasn't happening. But since it is, I'm here to sit next to you and hold your hand until the pain starts to lessen."

What if we didn't give everyone a participation trophy in an effort to teach the important lesson of defeat and disappointment, while simultaneously teaching the lessons of good sportsmanship and strong work ethic?

We are so focused on not allowing our kids and ourselves to experience pain. Instead, we do whatever it takes to get rid of the uncomfortable feelings immediately.

I get it! However, if we're honest with ourselves, this is not real life. It's a temporary "fix" to the problem, but it doesn't set anyone up for success down the road. The same goes with using food as a coping mechanism—it's a temporary "fix," but it doesn't serve anyone well in the long run.

I saw the effects of this firsthand when my girls participated in a dribble relay at halftime of a high school basketball game. My girls' team placed third, but only the first-place team got a medal. My girls cried all the way home—big, legitimate, puppy-dog tears—crying, "I don't understand why we didn't get a medal; everyone always gets a medal." It was a great opportunity for me to teach them a lesson on disappointment and how to be a gracious loser. Notice the story ended with a conversation rather than an ice cream cone, which would only have temporarily distracted them from their angst.

The Five S's of Mindful Eating Reviewed

Take a look at these five mindful eating tips and see which one resonates the most with you right now.

1. Sit down
2. Slow down
3. Simplify
4. Savor
5. Smile

Which one do you struggle with the most? Start there. Do not try to conquer everything at once, creating too many goals. That doesn't work and it can leave you feeling exhausted and disappointed.

Pick one S that you want to work on and just focus on that. If you forget, just pick up and start taking action the moment you remember—even if you only have two bites of your meal left. Each time you practice, it will get easier (kind of like training a muscle). Once you feel comfortable, move to the next S. There is no rush in this journey, because health is not a competition (thank goodness).

The whole point of these mindful eating tips is to be fully present during times of eating and help you identify patterns of behavior during emotional times. If you want to remember to do these five things in stress, then you must practice them in health. I guarantee you won't remember to sit down and smile when you're anxious just because you read about it in this book. You must use this practice every time you eat so that it becomes habit for the times you do use food as a coping mechanism. Over time, it will become easier to identify your emotions so you can deal with them in an appropriate manner.

My favorite word when it comes to health is "yet." We don't have to have it all figured out *yet*, but we do need to take one step toward (our goal). Being present during eating is absolutely a step toward health you won't regret.

repeat

The Kindness Challenge

Our emotions are a big part of our identities. They describe who we are and dictate our actions. Lately, I feel like the word "kindness" has been following me around. First, at an Enneagram workshop I attended a few months ago, the instructor mentioned that random acts of kindness light up the same reward centers in our brains as cocaine and sugar. Then, last Sunday, our pastor read the infamous line, "Love is patient, love is kind..." (1 Cor. 13:4).

I wrote those six words on a sticky note and placed it in our upstairs bathroom. The morning I wrote this entry, I was listening to a podcast and the host spoke about how kindness has a ripple effect, increasing serotonin levels in the person doing the kind act, in the person receiving the kind act, and in people witnessing the kind act. It's the perfect trifecta!

Serotonin is the hormone responsible for making us feel good. An imbalance of our serotonin levels can lead to a disruption in mood and increased chances of depression and anxiety.[2] From a nutrition standpoint, eating carbohydrates, which produces an insulin response and thereby binding to amino acids without tryptophan, can help free up tryptophan to cross the blood brain barrier, helping to create more serotonin (there's a little more to it but that's the overall gist). No wonder we call foods like mashed potatoes and macaroni and cheese comfort foods! They can help create more serotonin!

More times than not, the reason people overeat is emotional. It's a coping mechanism created to avoid dealing with the pain of the moment and can temporarily dull the internal feelings of being uncomfortable. Right or wrong, it works in the moment, which is why so many of us resort to this practice. What if random acts of kindness are the secret weapon to boosting your serotonin levels, which then allows you to feel better without grabbing the ice cream at night?

Who knew cleaning the snow off of a coworker's car would be the magic bullet to avoiding the drive-thru on the way home? What's even more amazing is if someone witnesses you cleaning the snow off the car, you could secretly be helping him or her avoid the drive-thru on the way home too!

Kindness is of the heart. It goes beyond being a nice person. It changes us and can lead to change in others. When I first started listening to all of this kindness talk, I initially dismissed it as a great idea that warrants too big a time commitment.

Then, I realized how utterly ridiculous that sounded. I was ashamed to have even thought it in the first place, because, isn't that why we're here on Earth? If I don't have the time to be kind, then this conversation better be a wakeup call to slow down and reprioritize how I allocate my time.

I invite you to create pockets of time in your day and look for opportunities to show kindness to others. In the morning, give a little forethought to the people you will encounter throughout the day. Then, come up with a kind gesture and follow through. After a while, you won't need to plan it out and will just naturally see the opportunities.

Write the note, pick up the phone and call instead of texting (and say something genuinely thoughtful while you're at it), spend the extra five minutes getting to know someone you would otherwise walk past, or hold the door open. Kind acts are often about the gift of time. Giving up your precious time shows other individuals you see them and that they matter. Think of the ripple effect we can create when we all choose to do life this way together. Who knows? Maybe your waistline will see the difference too.

choose your plan

Affirmation

Repeat this statement every day this week:

"I can do hard things."

Action

Before you consume a meal, ask yourself if you feel like smiling. If the answer is no, engage in some other activity (listen to music, call a friend, take a few breaths) until you feel better.

Achieve

Perform a random act of kindness every day this week.

Analyze

Think back to a time when you sat in your own "suckiness." What techniques did you use to get through the pain? How can you invite the pain instead of pretending it doesn't exist the next time you experience a difficult situation?

Accountability

Answer the below questions in your dedicated healthy lifestyle journal:

What change did you attempt to make this week?

Were you happy with the results?

What challenges did you encounter?

How would you do things differently next time?

5-star recipes
Chicken Noodle Soup

When life gives you lemons, make lemony chicken noodle soup. It's good for the body and soul and is comfort food at its finest.

Makes 8 servings

Ingredients

2 TBS olive oil

4 carrots, cut into bite-size pieces

3 stalks celery, chopped

1 large onion, chopped

2 cloves garlic, minced

½ tsp dried thyme

2 bay leaves

1½ tsp salt

¼ tsp pepper

2 lbs. chicken tenders, cut into bite-size pieces

12 cups low-sodium chicken broth

2 cups egg noodle pasta

3 TBS fresh lemon juice

1 cup fresh parsley, chopped

Directions

1. Heat the oil in a large pot or Dutch oven over medium heat. Add the carrots, celery, onion, garlic, thyme, bay leaves, salt, and pepper. Cook, stirring frequently, until the vegetables are soft, about 10 minutes.

2. Add chicken and broth to the pot. Bring to a boil, reduce heat, and simmer until the chicken is cooked through, approximately 15 minutes.

3. Add the noodles to the soup and cook until al dente, approximately 5 minutes. Add the lemon juice and parsley and stir to combine. Remove bay leaves and serve immediately.

Cannellini Chocolate Cake

Some people choose to show kindness through baked goods, so why not make a healthier version with protein and fiber? I promise the only thing people will taste in this recipe is rich, chocolaty goodness.

Makes 12 servings

Ingredients

1¼ cups semisweet chocolate chips
1 (15 oz.) can cannellini beans, rinsed and drained
2 tsp vanilla
4 eggs
½ cup sugar
½ tsp baking powder
1 TBS confectioners sugar, for dusting

Directions

1. Preheat oven to 350°F. Using nonstick cooking spray, grease and flour a 9-inch, round cake pan.
2. Pour chocolate chips into a heat-safe bowl. Bring medium pot of water to simmer and place bowl on top of pot to create a double broiler. Stir chocolate chips constantly until melted.
3. Combine the beans, vanilla, and eggs in the bowl of a food processor. Process until smooth. Next add sugar and baking powder, and continue to blend until all ingredients are incorporated.
4. Add the melted chocolate to food processer and blend until smooth.
5. Pour batter into the prepared cake pan. Bake for 40 minutes, or until a knife inserted into the center of the cake comes out clean.
6. Transfer cake to wire rack for 10 to 15 minutes before inverting onto a serving plate, or just save a dish and serve from the pan.
7. Sprinkle confectioners sugar just before serving.

Source: Adapted from Wellness Concepts[3]

lesson 12

It's Time to Set the Record Straight

"There is no elevator to success, you have to take the stairs."
—Zig Ziglar

We'll continue to do some heavy lifting as we add yet another layer to our foundation. No need to worry though, because I'll be with you the entire time. My job as a dietitian is not only to provide education, but also to get in the trenches with you. It's time we both got our boots a little muddy.

In order to do this nutrition thing right, we must clear the cobwebs of lies we have accepted as truths. I'll be the first to admit I believed a lot of them for a really long time. I thought holding onto these false truths were sources of motivation, but I learned they were holding me back from living my best life. I was missing out on the greatest gift I ever received, because my head told me otherwise.

Additionally, there are another set of lies we hear—ones told to us by manufacturing companies as to what constitutes as healthy. Marketing and advertising have us so confused as to what is fact and what is fiction. Now we believe Lucky Charms are healthy, because they are made with whole grains. We have traded logic for flair and it's time we take ourselves to nutrition school. Our best weapon of defense is the food label.

Finally, we discuss the three guiding nutrition principles every diet in America doesn't want you to know about. It may be the hardest concept to understand, but once you do, you will feel liberated rather than restricted.

nourish

Sanity over Thinness

By definition, cognitive dissonance is the state of having inconsistent thoughts, beliefs, or attitudes, especially as relating to behavioral decisions and attitude change.[1]

I simply call it "disconnect." Thankfully, it doesn't happen all too often in my mind, but when it does, it occupies all my time and energy. One area of disconnect I struggled with for a long time was feeling out of control whenever I tried to manage my weight.

Blogger and coach Isabel Foxen Duke helps dieters stop the binge eating/restrictive eating cycle. She does amazing work and is leading the charge on ending the war with food, helping us come to a place of sanity. She's a little brazen and outspoken, but she apologizes to no one and I like that about her. She is passionate about her work and it shows.

"I choose sanity over thinness every time," she said in a podcast.[2]

Wow. Let that sink in for a little.

I choose sanity over thinness every time.

It sounds like a good place to be mentally, but there is a certain comfort level around trying to manipulate your food choices to become a different size. I'll be honest, I love the concept, but the application of choosing sanity was a little too deep and scary for me to fully wrap my brain around. I assume people would expect that a dietitian wouldn't struggle with this, but this writing comes from a place of complete honesty. If we can't be authentic with one another, then what is our purpose?

My Experience With Food and Fashion

I have been preoccupied with my weight since I was in fourth grade when I started my first exercise group during recess. Instead of playing kickball, I was doing squats. I am so thankful I grew up in a small town where size and fashion were not a priority, because it probably would have taken me to another level of obsession.

It wasn't until I met Jim and moved to a more suburban area that I became aware of the judgmental eyes of others.

When Jim and I were first dating, we had just finished working out at the gym, and I decided to drive to the grocery store to pick up some food for dinner. I was still wearing my t-shirt and mesh shorts (reminder: mesh shorts were cool at one time) and grabbed my keys to walk out the door.

"Are you wearing that to the grocery store?" Jim questioned, stopping me in my tracks.

I looked down at my outfit. There were no visible stains, although I was sure I smelled a little bit.

"Sure," I shrugged my shoulders, confused where he was going with the conversation.

"What if you see someone you know?"

"Then I will stop and say 'Hi.' What is going on?"

"Nothing ... I just thought you would want to change first."

Toto, I've a feeling we're not in Lancaster County anymore.

Going to the grocery store in mesh shorts must be some sort of faux pas even though the thought was utterly ridiculous to me. Apparently, people would judge me by the clothes I wore in a supermarket, which told me that these folks had way too much time on their hands.

As a dietitian, I have become accustomed to the onceover shot my way whenever I meet someone new for the first time. It's done discreetly and mostly by other women, and I know exactly what they are asking themselves in that moment.

"Do I want to take advice from someone who looks this way?"

There is a certain level of pressure to look a certain way in the profession I chose. Let's be completely candid here. People don't feel comfortable taking advice from an overweight dietitian, because if she can't get it right, how can anyone expect to change? Let's just call it what it is instead of dancing around the issue.

I realize it's not the only profession facing this challenge. Personal trainers, speakers, actors, singers, executives, and medical professionals all have a "responsibility" to look a certain way. This self-perceived pressure has led me to my own cycles of restrictive eating and overeating in hopes of controlling my weight and fulfilling the standard appearance I think people demand.

Now you see the dilemma I'm facing. How am I supposed to heal people's relationships with food when I'm dealing with my own demons? How can I choose sanity over thinness every time when sanity may change the way my body looks and, therefore, possibly jeopardize my career? Am I being overdramatic with my thoughts? If fear of weight gain and sanity cannot coexist, then which one do I choose?

I wish I had clear answers to all of these questions, because I can imagine I am not the only one wrestling with these thoughts. Duke says healing cannot come with any expectations of a number. This means you can't find sanity if you are secretly hoping it will produce weight loss. You have to choose one.

Body acceptance is the first step to achieving sanity. Body acceptance is not the same as body love. Acceptance is simply choosing to say, "I accept the way my body looks just like I accept the fact the sky is blue." Again, another hard pill to swallow if you follow any social media feed or watch TV. The diet industry thrives on us feeling bad about our bodies and being desperate to make changes. Body love is not necessary for healing, although it will change your life for the better and improve confidence levels. Who doesn't need that?

Back to the question at hand: how do I heal someone's relationship with food—in other words, teach sanity—when I struggle with the same thing? By coaching people how to lose weight, am I feeding into the cycle that we desperately need to stop? Maybe Duke is wrong and this is a place where both can exist instead of one or the other. The question we have to ask is, what would that look like?

I frequently tell my patients you will never "arrive." If you don't like your body at 200 pounds, chances are you won't like your body at 150 pounds. We live in a society where "never enough" trumps contentment, just like the song in The Greatest Showman, "Never Enough." Rather than being about the destination, nutrition (like life) is about the journey. It is about what you learn and whom you help along the way. Those are your benchmarks.

I recently ran into my friend, Meg, at the YMCA. Meg is the ultimate source of encouragement and that's why I love her so much! She's extremely fit and she has a heart for Jesus, so we frequently talk about our lives and faith while running on the treadmill. I don't run into her too often, but when I do, I know she is a safe person to whom I can come with my own personal struggles and how they carry over into my practice. I asked, "How could I help others when I feel like I'm failing myself? Why do I have this need to be a certain number or look a certain way?"

Meg lovingly gazed at me and gently reminded me to seek my motivation.

"What is your purpose? What are you trying to accomplish? Who are you doing this for? Are you working so hard to gain more business so you can help others? Are you working so hard to make more money? Are you fulfilling your calling or do you have your own personal list of accomplishments you are trying to master?"

My answer, which I knew right away, was that I was making myself crazy for my own personal agenda. I was trying to hide it behind the lie that I was trying to look a certain way for my patients, when in reality I was still choosing thinness over sanity.

Don't get me wrong, I love helping people and I know it is my gift, but the craziness and added pressure I was putting on myself was not so I could be a better dietitian. It was so I could look good in a bathing suit. However, God isn't calling me to look good in a bathing suit. He couldn't care less about physical appearances. He is looking at my heart and asking me to be a good steward of the resources he gave me. Occupying my time and mental energy around food and weight was counterproductive to this particular calling.

I am happy to report that after months of hard work, I chose sanity. I can't say I am perfect in my execution every time and that those thoughts don't try to creep back in, but I'm working on it. Meg's advice was the prelude to a beautiful tale filled with surrender and acceptance. It shut down the insecurities imprisoning my self-worth and instead opened the door to freedom and a haven where I could take a deep breath and let my shoulders relax.

Declaring sanity allowed me to be the person God designed me to be, which feels amazing, invigorating, and peaceful all at the same time. Ultimately, it's my desire for you to feel those same feelings too.

eat

What's in Your Food?

We've all heard the catchy slogan from Capital One credit cards, "What's in your wallet?" Here, I bring it home and ask, "What's in your food?" Choosing simple, living ingredients as the base to your diet is an easy way to ensure you know the contents of your meals. There's no confusion about what's in a banana—the banana, itself, is the ingredient. It's the foods made up of multiple ingredients that get a little trickier.

In our practice, we teach people how to read a food label. There are seven fundamental tips I teach my clients on how to decipher whether a food is a diet staple or an every-once-in-a-while food. Notice, I didn't categorize foods as good or bad, because there is no such thing. Any diet that tells you otherwise may be ill-advised.

There are foods that are more nutrient dense (more nutrients than calories) and foods more energy dense (more calories than nutrients), but each food has its time and place to be fully enjoyed. Obviously, the more nutrient-dense foods you select, the better you will feel. I always encourage my patients to eat foods that rot, because if the food rots, then it means it has life in the form of vitamins and minerals.

Look at it this way: your body is constantly changing. Every four weeks, you make new skin cells, and every three months, you make new red blood cells. Where do you get the raw materials to make those new cells? Your food! If you put good, healthy, nutritious foods into your body, you will have healthy cells that provide energy, mental clarity, and focus. If you put dead, chemical junk into your body, you will create cells that are depleted and sluggish.

Think of a carpenter. If he wants to make a strong dining room table, will he choose oak or particleboard? No contest, oak is strong, sturdy, and built to last. The same holds true with our bodies.

The Food Label: Seven Keys to Success

At the time of publication, the new nutrition labels have yet to be released, although we are starting to see more and more labels bearing the new style. Before looking at the nutrition facts and ingredient list of a given label, it's always important to check out the serving size and servings per container. If you skip out on this part, you may mistake four servings for one. I met with a patient today who ate half of a frozen pizza. She showed me, with her hands, how big the pizza was. It appeared to be a single serving pizza. However, when we looked up the nutrition label, the serving size was one-third of the pizza. Had she eaten the whole pizza, she would have consumed well over 1,000 calories. Her assumption that the serving size was half of the pizza was incorrect.

Let's dive into seven key places to look on a food label so you can achieve the highest level of success in your dietary goals.

First, **fiber** fills you up without having to eat a ton of it. While it has many health benefits, the amount of fiber we consume doesn't add up quickly, so aim to look for products with 3 grams of fiber or more per serving. The recommended daily goal for women is 25 grams of fiber per day and for men is 38 grams of fiber per day. Choosing whole grains, beans, nuts, seeds, fruits, and vegetables as the base of your diet will get you to this number. Always be sure to increase fiber slowly and with plenty of water.

Second, whenever possible, **choose whole grains** over enriched. Long story short, enriched means "synthetically adulterated." During modern refining processes, the outer bran layer and germ are stripped from the endosperm to create a smooth consistency. Unfortunately, these two layers are where all the fiber and B-vitamins are contained. Stripping these layers means stripping the food of most of its nutrition. Sure, we have a nice, smooth texture, but the grain is void of nutrients.

How do refined grains get their nutritional value back up to par? By a process known as enrichment, which means the nutrients that were once there, but lost to processing, are added back in synthetically. Typically, enriched products do not contain as much fiber and nutrients as their whole grain counterparts. There are also arguments as to whether our bodies absorb synthetic vitamins in the same way as those occurring naturally in foods.

Third, **sugar** is found in everything. It makes products taste better, so manufacturers would be remiss to overlook an opportunity to intensify flavor. I once read that an average person in the mid-1700s consumed five pounds of sugar per year, whereas in 2012, the average person consumed three pounds of sugar per week.[3] Given the latter statistic, an average person will consume an industrial-sized dumpster's worth of sugar in his or her lifetime. The recommendations for sugar intake for women are less than 24 grams of added sugar per day and less than 36 grams of added sugar per day for men. It's important to note these recommendations are based on added grams, meaning, "added by the manufacturer." Natural sugars (found in foods, such as fruits, vegetables, and plain dairy products) are exempt from this recommendation. When the new nutrition labels are fully in effect, ca. 2020, it will be a lot easier to distinguish added sugars from natural sugars. Until then, we have to do our best to calculate them by looking to see where sugar falls on the ingredient list. Since ingredients are listed from most to least by weight, the higher sugar falls on the list, the more likely the source is coming from the manufacturer. Also take note that food companies can be sneaky and may use different sources of sugar instead of one type. Using a bunch of different sugars in small amounts keeps sugar farther down the list. Some cereals may list six different types of sugar.

When it comes to sugar, you are in charge of how you want to spend your daily allotment. Think of me as your banker giving you money to spend. If talking to a woman, I will give her the following options: you may want to spend your entire $24 on one, big-ticket item, or spread it out between a few, smaller-priced options. Either decision is fine. The only rule is, you cannot save your money to spend tomorrow. You get a fresh $24 each day, but it never rolls over if unused. You can choose to spend all of it, none of it, or some of it. The beauty is, you get to make the right decision for you. I once had a patient who told me on her first visit that if I try to take chocolate away, she would not be successful. Not a problem! We found out her daily intake included roughly 12 grams of added sugar through the products she was eating. That left 12 grams remaining! We calculated one Hershey kiss to be 3 grams of sugar, which meant she could eat four kisses through her daily diet each day if she wished. I'm happy to report she is one of my most successful clients. She found a middle ground she could sustain while meeting her health goals.

Fourth, **avoid the words high fructose corn syrup**. In short, high fructose corn syrup (HFCS) is a highly processed sugar that not only impacts blood sugars dramatically, but in some cases, has also been found to mess with the body's fullness signals. Anything that messes with your ability to determine fullness is a big "no, thank you" in my book.

Fifth, when it comes to **fat**, we need some in our diet, despite the negative connotation it gets from time to time. Thirty percent of our caloric intake should come from fat, but sadly, the standard American diet typically contains a lot more due to an increase in individuals eating out and consuming processed foods. Since the goal is 30 percent of your total intake, one easy way to look at a food to determine healthfulness is to apply the "3 grams per 100 calories" rule. For every 100 calories a food provides, up to 3 grams of fat is acceptable (ex. 200 calories: up to 6 grams acceptable, 300 calories: up to 9 grams acceptable, and so on and so forth). By no means do I want you breaking out the calculator in the middle of the grocery aisle trying to micromanage the situation. Simply use it as a means to compare products. If a particular food item is 245 calories and has 8 grams of fat, I say close enough. However, if that same food has 14 grams of fat, I would suggest looking into other options.

Sixth, **avoid partially hydrogenated oils**. This is a fancy way of saying avoid trans fats. Unfortunately, manufacturers can add up to a half a gram of this unhealthy fat into a food product without having to list it on the nutrient facts label. Since most of us consume more than one serving of the products we eat, there's a good chance we are eating 1 or 2 grams of trans fats without even realizing it. I generally teach patients to glance over the trans fat section of the label without putting much faith into the number and instead focus on whether or not the words "partially hydrogenated oils" are present. If you see those words, quickly put the product down and back away slowly. Since most trans fats have been removed from products, you may not see too many of these sinister words anymore. I still see them from time to time on the back of a peanut butter label. Choosing natural versions of nut butters will help ensure a trans-fat-free experience.

Finally, number seven on the list concerns **sodium**, one of those minerals that can greatly impact our blood pressure and kidney function. Chances are, if we all lived to the ripe, old age of 100, we would all have high blood pressure. It's a natural part of aging. Eating a high-sodium diet can expedite that process. Again, processed foods and dining out frequently can all add a boatload of salt to our diets. Most people challenge this by telling me they don't use the saltshaker, so they should be good to go. Unfortunately, 90 percent of our sodium doesn't come from the saltshaker; rather it comes from the foods we select. The daily recommendations for sodium are no more than 2,300 milligrams per day, which is roughly 1 teaspoon, unless you're middle aged, of African American descent, or have a history of high blood pressure; then that recommendation goes down to 1,500 milligrams per day. Aim to look for products with roughly 250 milligrams or less per serving to stay within the guidelines above. Another easy guideline is to follow the "5:20 rule." When looking at the %Daily Values (based on an average, 2,000-calorie diet), anything with a 5 percent or lower %Daily Value is considered low and anything with 20 percent or higher %Daily Value is considered high. Honestly, the only thing you want high on that food label is fiber. Everything else is best lower. Anything between 5 and 20 percent is at your discretion and will need to be balanced with other items in your diet.

So, there you have it—a quick guide to label reading. It is important to note: please **do not** try to conquer the grocery store all at once. It is too much information and you will end up ditching your cart by aisle two. Go home, open your pantry and fridge, and see what baby step will work for you right now. If the products in your house already are in line with the above guidelines, great! No need to make any changes. However, if a product falls outside the recommendations, next time you're at the grocery store, spend a few moments comparing products and slowly begin to transition your inventory. Most importantly, I want to give you the tools to be successful. Now you can shop with authority and confidence!

repeat
The Three Crucial Steps to a Healthy Life

If you were to ask someone at the American Dietetic Association to define a healthy diet in three words, he or she would probably use the words "variety, balance, and moderation." Those were the three words I wrote at the top of my notebook when I took my first nutrition class. When I tell my clients to use these three words as their guiding principles to a healthy lifestyle, I typically get a confused look.

"Where's the list of rules? Where are the listings of foods I can only eat or need to avoid? What do you mean I can still eat chocolate if I want? I don't understand what these three foreign words mean!"

We have been conditioned to the idea of dieting looking one, specific way. No matter the diet—Keto, Paleo, Isagenix, intermittent fasting—we are taught there are rules to follow and not be broken. If we want results (let's be real, no one is doing this just for fun), we have to perform everything as written in the bylaws. The rules are not negotiable. You are either following them and succeeding or breaking them and failing. There is no wiggle room or gray areas, because everything is black or white.

So, when I start to introduce "gray" words like "balance, variety, and moderation," it's natural to get a confused reaction from the masses. When my clients first come in, they want black and white, because that is all they know from past experience. New territory is always scary and confusing.

So, let's dive into the meaning of these three words a bit more in terms of your diet and provide some clarification.

Variety means just that; you need to eat more than three foods. In the beginning, when we try a new diet, it is common for clients to eat similar foods, because there is safety in knowing exactly what the macronutrient distribution is and how the food will make them feel. Eventually, though, they will get bored, and when they do, they tend to seek out exciting (and often high-calorie) alternatives.

My advice to patients is to try one or two new foods and/or recipes every one to two weeks. It never fails, though, as I always have those few patients who insist they can eat the same foods day in and day out and not get bored.

I was working with a guy who promised me for months he was happy as can be eating similar foods. Then, all of a sudden, he wasn't. He told his partner if he has to eat chicken and green beans one more time, he's leaving and not coming back.

Boredom is one reason to embrace variety, but you should also understand variety's importance in maximizing the body's ability to receive diverse nutrients. If you eat the same three foods over and over again, chances are you are missing out on some key vitamins and minerals necessary for your body to work optimally. When your body is deficient in key nutrients, you may actually experience more intense cravings, as your body is trying to get you to eat them through your food. Intense cravings and dieting never end well. Eating fruits and vegetables seasonally is just one way to ensure variety in your diet.

Balance is defined as, "a state in which different things occur in equal or proper amounts or have an equal or proper amount of importance," according to Merriam-Webster.[4] Visualize a balance beam. As you try to walk across to the other side, with your hands out to your side to help reinforce balance, it is fairly easy to walk across the narrow beam, because your palms are empty. Let's add a 10-pound dumbbell to one palm. Your body has to work a little harder to accommodate for the imbalance. You may throw your hip out to the side to stabilize, but let's be honest, throwing your hip out to the side over time can lead to lower back pain.

What if you add eating takeout three times a week to your routine, which means less cooking and less overall vegetable intake, and now try to walk across the beam? All of a sudden, you may notice weight gain, which makes walking across that beam harder.

In addition to takeout, you now add impaired immune system to the equation due to the lack of key nutrients in your diet. You begin to contract common colds more frequently resulting in your body being exhausted and needing extra sleep. It's amazing for you to take one step without toppling over.

Balance means equal amounts. It also means equal amounts when you are on vacation. Most people view vacations as a time to do whatever they want and face the consequences when they return home. They throw balance right out the window.

Jim and I recently went on a kids-free vacation to Colorado to celebrate our 15-year anniversary. We knew we wanted to be active, but also wanted to try local fare and breweries. We saw a barbecue place with the line wrapped around the building while we were driving one day. Since the restaurant was off the main street, we figured this must be where all the locals went for some good food. Barbecue isn't exactly nutritious, but it sure is tasty. So, in order to visit the restaurant that evening, we ate a big salad for lunch. We split our barbecue dinner platter since the portions were so large. We didn't tell ourselves we couldn't eat high-calorie food, we just found balance to make it work.

Finally, we come to **moderation**. To me, this means, "not too much or too often." Webster defines it as, "avoiding extremes or excesses."[5] Notice it does not use the word "never." When we use the word "never," we are back to following rules.

"Moderation" is extremely confusing, because *what is* too much or too often? The truth is, every person's definition of too much or too often will be different. For some, "not too often" means yearly, while for others, it could mean once per month.

Most diets will tell you to follow an "80/20 rule." If you're eating well 80 percent of the time, then you can splurge 20 percent of the time. This usually works great for those practicing maintenance (not trying to gain or lose any

157

weight). Depending on where you are in your health journey, this may be a great starting place for you too. Again, it's different for each person. The bottom line is, you have to ask yourself if your definition of moderation is getting you closer or further away from your health goals. Obviously, if it is taking you further away, you may need to tighten things up and decrease the frequency of certain habits or vices.

Stop Following Rules or Create New Ones

I'm a rule follower. I am a first-born, straight-A student who has a gift for identifying what people are seeking and then delivering. Rules don't scare me; they excite me. I am fueled by "a job well done" and gold stars. Growing up, dieting was a challenge I was excited to conquer. I enjoyed writing New Year's Resolutions and filling out notebooks and spreadsheets of workouts and calorie intake at the beginning of any program I started.

As with anything, though, reality sets in. I got busy. Motivation went out the window. I just wanted a cookie. The minute my pristine notebook no longer followed the rules, I quit. In fact, I didn't just quit. I ran the other direction. The panic I felt in my chest and the loathing I had for myself felt like a lump in my gut, and it was overwhelming. So, I ate.

My eating left me feeling so uncomfortable I wanted to hide and cry. I suppose I was trying to punish myself for messing up. It didn't work. It had the opposite effect. Instead of changing my behavior, I ended up gaining weight.

When I was younger, taking tennis lessons, every time I messed up a forehand shot, I hit the side of my leg with my racket to punish myself. That didn't work either. It just made my leg hurt, which impeded my ability to get to the ball. I finally got to a point where I realized my technique was wrong. You see, shame and pain never motivate, but treating your body kindly does. I had to change my technique.

If years of striving for perfection proved not to be the answer, then what if I tried the opposite? What if instead of following rules, I stopped creating them? What if I used words like variety, balance, and moderation in an honest, integrity-filled way and simply applied them to my life?

I gave it a shot, supplying my body with a variety of foods to eat without any rules attached. I fed my body foods that both were tasty and sustained my fullness. I balanced fun treats with low-calorie salads, not to stay within a certain calorie range, but because that is what my body craved.

I now happily accept the Sonic Blast my husband buys me on his way home from work and share it with my kids instead of eating all of it after everyone has gone to bed.

Envisioning myself standing on a balance beam with my arms out-stretched, I ask myself at the end of most days, "Have I remained upright without overcompensating in any one direction?" I'm still strategically listening for those words "job well done," but I'm finding these are the victories I actually crave. Even though I'm wired for rules, I realize I'm wired for them short-term, but the race I'm running in this lifetime is for the duration.

Don't get me wrong. The dazzling lights and bright colors each new, fad diet promises can easily distract me. I've had enough practice over the years to be able to identify those shiny diets for what they are and can stay true to my course. If your story looks anything like mine, I invite you to try a different way too.

Understanding variety, balance, and moderation, and using them as guidelines as opposed to following a list of rules, will ultimately help you reach your goals, both short-term and for the rest of your life. Remember, the goal is not to stay on this weight-loss/weight-gain yo-yo for the rest of our lives. It is about doing the hard work up front and reaping the benefits for years and years, instead of taking the quick fix route that leaves us feeling depressed, defeated, and at a higher weight than we started six to twelve months prior.

Michael Pollan in his book, *In Defense of Foods*, summed up a healthy diet in seven words: "Eat food, mostly plants, not too much."[6] Looks like he took the same nutrition class I did and wrote the same three words at the top of his page!

choose your plan

Affirmation

Repeat this statement every day this week:

"I choose sanity over thinness every time."

Action

Try a new recipe this week.

Achieve

Use the page from Appendix B as a cheat sheet to help navigate whether the products you purchase at your grocery store are an everyday staple or an every-once-in-a-while splurge.

Analyze

Tonight, as you prepare to go to bed, imagine yourself standing on a balance beam. Did your choices keep you standing tall or leaning too far to one side? How can you make adjustments tomorrow to bring a different outcome? Write it down in your journal and read your thoughts tomorrow as a reminder of what steps to take to keep you progressing toward your goals

Accountability

Answer the below questions in your dedicated healthy lifestyle journal:

What change did you attempt to make this week?

Were you happy with the results?

What challenges did you encounter?

How would you do things differently next time?

5-star recipes
Fruit and Spinach Salad

*My friend, Kristin, made me this salad when I came home from the hospital after having the twins. This salad is great for brunch and entertaining. It's the perfect **balance** of sweet and savory.*

Servings can be adjusted based on volume of ingredients used

Ingredients

For the Salad
   Spinach
   Banana, sliced
   Canned Mandarin oranges, drained
   Strawberries, sliced
   Pecans & Feta cheese (optional)
For the Dressing
   ¼ cup sugar
   ½ cup olive oil
   ⅓ cup white vinegar
   1 TBS chopped onion
   1 TBS poppyseeds
   ¼ tsp salt

Directions

1. Prepare the salad by combining all ingredients in a large bowl.
2. Combine all dressing ingredients in a Mason jar (or any container with a lid). Shake until incorporated and pour desired amount onto your salad. Mix well.

Power Burgers

Eating a greasy burger can have you leaning sideways on a balance beam, but making your own and swapping in healthier ingredients will have you standing tall and proud in no time. Try this tasty dish from my colleague Kristen and check out her website below for other healthy creations.

Makes 4 servings

Ingredients

1 pound ground chicken or turkey
1 egg
⅓ cup raw steel-cut oats
1 TBS chia seeds
1 tsp red pepper flakes
1 tsp garlic powder
1 tsp onion powder
Salt and pepper to taste

Directions

1. Preheat oven to 350°F and spray sheet pan with non-stick spray.
2. Mix all ingredients listed above together.
3. Form into four patties, place on sheet pan.
4. Bake in oven for 25 minutes.
5. Assemble your burger and enjoy!

Source: Kristen Peterson, MPH, RDN, LDN, PrimeLifeNutrition.org[7]

lesson 13

The Unspeakable Truth

*"If you think the pursuit of good health is expensive
and time consuming, try illness."*
—*Lee Swanson*

I have seen so many retired (and on-the-verge-of-retiring) individuals in my office with hopes and dreams of travel and time off, only to be handed medical diagnoses requiring frequent doctor visits, testing, and medications. The picturesque vision of a perfect retirement—golf games in the afternoon and social dinners at night—soon are met with the reality of lifestyle changes and activity restrictions.

I once had a patient whose doctor told her if she can make it through her 60s with minimal medical issues, then she's got smooth sailing in her remaining years. Apparently, our 60s are a decade in which the decisions we've made in our younger years finally catch up with us. Unfortunately, I have been seeing earlier arrivals as poor lifestyle changes are catching victims earlier.

Obviously, I don't have a crystal ball, so I cannot predict who will need medical intervention and who will not. What I do know is there are some guiding principles that, if executed properly, will put us at a major advantage. As always, some of these are mental and others are tangible and physical in nature. We will tackle them all with practical tips, accessible tools, and scientific recommendations.

I will warn you now: I'm going to talk about poop.

nourish

'I Didn't Know I Needed Shoes'

A few years ago, a librarian at one of the elementary schools in our school district asked me to be a guest on her TV show through the local school district channel. She received a grant to provide health information through video and thought it would be fun to create an episode where I show kids and their parents healthy, afterschool snack ideas. It sounded like a new adventure, so I agreed, despite finding the whole situation extremely nerve racking.

The show ended up a success and the producer asked if I would like to have my own nutrition show on the network. I felt like it was a great opportunity to help more people, so I agreed and ended up naming the show after our company, since creativity isn't always my thing and for a lack of any other ideas. To date, I have taped more than 20 shows and am finally starting to get more comfortable in front of a camera.

I end each episode with a cooking demonstration, and let me tell you, I have a newfound respect for cooking personalities on TV. It is extremely difficult to think, talk, and cook at the same time. In almost every episode, I end up spilling something!

A few months ago, I was scheduled to tape a show in my kitchen that taught viewers how to lighten up high-calorie breakfast recipes. It was going to be the first of a three-part series highlighting breakfast, lunch, and dinner recipes. Because of time commitments on the producer's end, we only had 90 minutes to shoot the video. We calculated this would be more than enough time to tape a 30-minute segment. The plan was for them to get to my house at noon to start setting up cameras and get right down to business at 12:30.

My twins went to afternoon kindergarten, so the bus picked them up outside my house at 12:28. We always walk out of the door at 12:26, which gives us plenty of time to walk down the driveway and exchange hugs and kisses with time to spare. Being a Type A personality, I'm a bit of a control freak when it comes to being places on time (thanks also to my dad). Nothing gives me more anxiety than being late.

Because the timing of the taping intertwined so closely with the girls' departure time, I had everything planned down to the minute.

The plan was to feed the girls lunch before the crew arrived and have them completely ready for school. One of the dishes I was lightening up was a cheese omelet, so I needed to make the high-calorie version right before we started taping so it wouldn't look waxy on the plate when I used it as a comparison. So far, things were going right as planned.

The guys got to my house at noon and immediately got to work setting everything up. I started cooking the food for the show while the girls were playing with their karaoke machine in the playroom. Every so often I yelled out to the girls, "we're leaving in seven minutes," or, "five more minutes girls, are you sure you're ready to go?"

Each time I was met with, "yes, mom," and I secretly congratulated myself for rocking the supermom title. I looked up at the clock on the stove and it finally read 12:26. I took the eggs off the burner and directed, "Girls, it's time to go!"

I walked out of the kitchen and into the living room. Remember, we live in an old farmhouse, which means no open floor plan. Chip and Joanna Gaines would have a field day at my house! Much to my surprise, the girls were nowhere to be found. I called their names louder, but still got no response. Did they go outside when the guys were walking in and out of my house?

I ran outside and started frantically screaming their names.

"Charley, Bella, this is not funny!"

Nothing. I ran back in the house and there was Bella, standing in the living room.

"Bella, where were you?" I rushed. "Nevermind. Where is your backpack? "It's time to go!"

"I don't know," she said, innocently.

"What do you mean you don't know? You just had it!"

"Oh, I hung it back up in the laundry room," she remembered.

"Okay, you go outside and stay on the porch," I instructed. "I'll get your backpack. Where is your sister?"

All of a sudden, there was Charley, casually strolling out of the playroom. Did they not hear me yelling their names? I was so tensely confused as to why no one understood the plan. No one was sticking to the plan!

"Charley, what are you doing?" seemingly repeating myself, "It's time to go!"

That's when I noticed she didn't have any shoes on.

"Charley, where are your shoes?!"

"I don't know," she said, the innocence starting to wear thin. "I must have taken them off."

"What do you mean, 'taken them off'?!"

I may have been screaming at this point.

"We don't have time to miss the bus today," I pleaded. "You have to get on

165

that bus. Mommy needs to start filming right after you leave. I want you to go upstairs and grab any two shoes you can find. I don't care if they match or if they are for the same foot. Just run as fast as you can and grab some shoes while I go grab your backpacks."

Charley, a 5-year-old kindergartner with no concept of time, went up our two flights of stairs to get to her room, as I was unable to refrain from complete panic. I ran through the kitchen to the laundry room, grabbed the backpacks that mysteriously got hung back up, all the while screaming like a crazy woman for Charley to hurry up.

When I walked out the front door to meet Bella, I saw the bus coming to a stop outside of my house. I began to tell Bella to run to the bus, but then realized I couldn't send just one kid. I needed them both, so I told Bella to stay with me. I looked back up at the house again, but saw no signs of Charley.

Amidst the chaos, a few cars started to line up behind the bus. I love my bus driver, but the look she gave me in that moment told me that she could no longer wait. I honestly couldn't even tell if Charley had made it to the third floor yet. So, the bus left. The day the girls absolutely could not miss the bus became the day they missed the bus.

As if scripted in a movie, Charley walked out of the house holding two shoes, and to her credit, she did find a matching pair. Standing in the driveway, I was completely dumbfounded about what to do next. The school wouldn't open its doors for another 20 minutes. If I waited, we would never have enough time to shoot the video. So, I did the only thing I knew with absolute certainty I could do … I started crying.

Seeing me cry, Charley immediately burst into tears of her own.

"I'm sorry, mommy, I'm sorry," she wailed. "I didn't know! I didn't know!"

"You didn't know what?" I cried back. "You didn't know you needed shoes? You always need shoes for school, honey. Today is no different than any other day. You always need shoes for school."

After a few seconds of complete and utter confusion, I pulled it together and figured out a plan. My friend, Lauren, who lives down the street, has a son that rode the same bus as my girls, but he wasn't picked up until 12:45. I decided to drive the girls to her house, hoping she could put the girls on the bus at her son's stop.

The girls had strict marching orders to get into the minivan while I ran inside to grab my keys. While I was inside, I asked the crew if there was any chance they heard my hysterics in the driveway. Smart guys—they told me they hadn't heard a thing.

Without any shoes of my own on, I told the crew I'd be back in five minutes and ran out the door. I was a sweaty mess from running around. Typically, I try to look nice for a taping, spending some extra time on my hair and makeup, but that day my viewers were in for a treat and got to see me as a mother of five, stringy hair and all.

I called Lauren on the way to let her know I was coming and that I would explain everything later. When I arrived at her house, she ran out the door and was exactly what my kids needed in that moment. I opened the van doors before the vehicle had even come to a full stop, yelling at the girls to get out of the car, and then proceeded to throw their backpacks and shoes on Lauren's front lawn.

Lauren didn't miss a beat. She hugged my girls and told them in a nice, calm, soothing voice how happy she was that she got to put them on the bus. I was so thankful for everything she did that day, because I was not winning any awards for my performance. As soon as I returned to the house, Andrew, the producer, handed me my microphone to attach to my shirt.

"How do I look?" I asked him, thinking I probably should have taken a couple seconds to look in a mirror. However, at that point, I was attached to the microphone and there was no more time to spare. I took a few breaths and we began to tape.

The Planning Paradox

Although the exact specifics may be different, the theme of this story will sound familiar to many other mothers in one way or another. Sometimes we can have everything planned down to the minute, but I'm learning that the more I try to control my life, the more God decides to have a sense of humor and teach me a lesson otherwise.

The same goes with dieting. The more we try to restrict our calories and control our exercise, the more things start to unravel, and the more out of control we may feel. It's quite the paradox.

The Philadelphia Eagles won the Super Bowl for the first time ever just a few weeks before I wrote this lesson. I was not the cool mom who took her kids out of school to go see the parade, because large crowds and traffic with lots of kids didn't sound like fun to me. Furthermore, because I'm that Type A, control freak, if we had decided to go, I would have had everyone up and out of the house at 3:45 a.m. to make sure we didn't hit any traffic and get the best view possible. After all, if we were going to go to Philly, I was going to make sure we had the best experience, regardless of the freezing weather and lack of clean bathroom facilities.

I was talking to a coworker who did make it to the parade and she had quite a different experience from the one I would have created. She went down with her dad just to be part of the experience. They left around 7 a.m. and had no problems finding a seat on a bus that left from a nearby town. They got a great spot on the parade route with a good view of the players as they rode by on a bus. The best part was that they were outside a building with restrooms and real plumbing! She said they had such a nice time being part of the celebration.

Hmmm ... sounds like she had a much better time than the one I would have tried to create while trying to control everything. Her lack of stress and carefree attitude allowed her and her dad to have a great experience together and create memories. I would have created memories too; they just would have been chaotic ones that you'd be reading about in the next lesson.

Sometimes we get so caught up trying to create the perfect experience— or follow the perfect diet—that we miss the bigger picture. We miss celebrating with our loved ones or enjoying the special moments, because we are obsessing over what we will eat, or not eat.

Where are some areas you can let go of your controlling tendencies with your diet? What moments are you missing out on because you are worried about calories? When it comes to your weight, one meal isn't going to radically alter the course of your diet. One piece of cake will not make you gain weight much in the same way one salad won't make you lose weight. It's all about balance. It's not an "either or" situation; rather, there can be room for both.

On my kids' birthdays, they will always remember me eating a piece of cake with them to help celebrate, and, if they think about it a little harder, they may also recall a big salad served with dinner. Creating balance is essential to long-term success. How can you create more balance in your own eating habits?

eat

Code Brown

Everyone knows that when you have babies you are going to have to change poopy diapers. You may have seen countless videos online of fathers gagging and trying their hardest not to let any trace of feces touch their hands. My husband was no different and always muttered plenty of comments, such as, "This is nasty," or, "This is so disgusting," or, "Ugh, the smell." He used to use half the wipes container on one diaper change. You can imagine how many wipes we went through in this house.

The worst part of changing diapers were the blowouts, where the poop would escape the top of the diaper and smear all over the baby's back. Pulling the onesie over the child's head without getting poop in his or her hair was a 50-percent success rate. It was much easier if Jim was home to help, but most of the time, my children decided to have these episodes when I was flying solo. I only found out years after the twins were out of diapers that onesies have their unique shoulder fold so you can pull it off by sliding the material *down* their bodies. That information would have been so helpful—oh I don't know—**five** babies ago!

On one rare occasion, Jim was home alone and one of the babies pooped through his diaper and shorts and all over the infant car seat. When I got home from wherever I was (let's face it, it was either work or the grocery store), I found the infant seat outside by the trashcan. When I questioned Jim about what had happened, he told me he didn't want to talk about it and I had permission to buy a new car seat.

These stories are not any different than most people's experiences with babies and pooping. It's when the kids get a little older that more challenges arise.

One boy refused to go number two, because he was afraid it would hurt (therefore making it hurt). I physically remember crying on the bathroom floor with him, begging him to just go, praying for wisdom, and feeling so hopeless.

Another child went almost three weeks without pooping. We were scared there was a blockage. When we got x-rays, the doctor diagnosed him with FOS (full of shit)! A couple enemas later and we were on our way.

Nothing tops the girls' experiences. I'm guessing they were around 15 months or so when they discovered they could reach into their diapers and smear poop all over their cribs, bedding, and the walls. This became a new, fun game to play after they woke up in the morning or from naps in the afternoon.

The bedroom was a warzone patrolled by two, quiet, sneaky little soldiers. I never heard anything on the monitor that would lead me to believe they were doing such a thing. It's nasty enough when one kid does this horrific act, but the stench of two kids' poop smearing can almost knock you out.

I asked around for advice on how to stop this insanity. The first thing we did was put their footed pajamas on backwards so they couldn't unzip them from the front. Problem solved, or so we thought. It worked for a day or two until they figured out how to pull their arms out of the sleeves and reach back to grab inside their diapers.

Jim had the bright idea of using packing tape! Every afternoon before naps and every night before bedtime, we put their pajamas on backwards and then made them put their hands up in the air, telling them they were under arrest. Next, we proceeded to put tape under their armpits and around their torsos so they couldn't pull their arms out of their sleeves. Finally, crisis averted, or so we thought. Those girls were always one step ahead of us. We later found them hopping into each other's crib to pull the tape off each other. I do admire their determination.

Our last, and thankfully, successful attempt was to add a final piece of clothing—pajamas backward, packing tape around the torso, and a pajama nightgown over top. After two months of battle, the parents won the war, exhausted from all the work involved getting them ready for bed!

Your Poop Tells a Story

Looking back on those stories, we can finally laugh, but pooping issues can be really serious. At every initial appointment, I have my patients look at a Bristol Stool Scale to show me what their "normal" poop looks like. (Google Bristol Stool Scale images right now to see where your normal falls on the list). It always makes the grown men squirm, but I remind them that their poop tells a story. I can easily identify deficits in hydration, fiber intake, and potential food intolerances, just by looking at which image they point to on the scale.

Fiber is one of the most important nutrients lacking in the Standard American Diet (unfortunately, the acronym SAD is pretty accurate). Fiber is only found in plant products, but we are starting to see more and more fiber added to products, such as yogurt, to enhance nutrient intake.

Foods that naturally contain fiber are fruits, vegetables, whole grains, beans, nuts, and seeds. Women should aim to consume 25 grams per day and men's fiber goal is 38 grams per day. I always suggest getting a baseline of a patient's current fiber intake before starting to add more.

Most Americans consume about 16 grams of fiber per day.[1] Pair that with low water intake and you have the perfect recipe for constipation.

When you do add more fiber into your diet, do so slowly and with the addition of lots of water. Add three to four grams every three to four days until you reach your goal instead of all at once. Doing it all at once is not a good idea, because your body will naturally revolt. I saw this firsthand in a patient who went from 15 grams on average to 50 grams overnight. She told me at her follow up visit that she had driven herself to the emergency room with terrible stomach cramps. The doctors diagnosed her with too much fiber. I asked her what made her add so much so quickly (against my advice) to which she responded she thought her body could handle it. Unfortunately, she learned the hard way that it could not. Learn from her. Don't do this.

Fiber's benefits exceed just keeping you regular. It can help control blood sugar, cholesterol, and bowel diseases, such as diverticulosis and colon cancer. Our intestinal systems are lined with trillions of bacterial cells. Their main job is to keep invaders out and to protect our body's health. These healthy bacteria feed on fiber. Let's keep them happy and thriving so they can do their job well.

Fiber also has this amazing ability to make you feel full for long periods of time. When it comes to weight management, fiber is your friend. There's nothing worse than trying to lose weight while feeling hungry. Those types of diets rarely work long term and can end up leaving you feeling depleted, or worse, consuming more calories through overeating.

Aim to get the recommended amount of fiber each day by choosing lots of fruits, veggies, beans, and whole grains. Eat the skin of produce and choose products with 100 percent whole grains or stone ground over enriched. Take notice how much healthier your body feels.

Finally, if you're in that stage where you're changing diapers, hang in there! There is a light at the end of the tunnel. Just make sure you have plenty of wipes and pull the onesie down.

repeat
Parent-Teacher Conferences

I realize not every parent enjoys parent-teacher conferences, but this particular day of the year is my Christmas. It's the one day of the year that I feel validated, supported, loved, and admired for my role as a mother.

Of course, I have to brag for just a moment—bear with me.

I have great kids. They act crazy at home, but apparently, they pull it together in the classroom. I'm so proud of each of them.

Jake is a hard worker and surpassing all expectations. Parker is a joy to have in class and is so kind and helpful. Charley is raising her hand and answering questions, out loud! She loves school. Bella is social, making lots of friends! This is huge considering the selective mutism testing fiasco you will learn about in Lesson 15.

The icing on the cake was Ben's teacher's comment: "He is such a quiet gentleman!" I nearly fell out of my chair and literally laughed out loud in the teacher's face. Of course, he is. He is the smart one and I tell him this every ... single ... day. I want this to become his inner voice instead of all the times I'm yelling at him about his poor choices.

Parent-teacher conferences are an opportunity for teachers to let us know how our children are doing when we're not there to watch over them. I give teachers so much credit. Not only do they manage to get all those children to listen and perform the same activity, but they also teach them new things that the children retain. I'm still not sure how they do this, because I have told my kids at least five gazillion times to hang their coats and backpacks up when they come through the door after school. At school they listen. At home, apparently, the rules are different.

Of course, it's easier to do things when you have a teacher working beside you day in and day out. After all, that's why people come to see me in my office. I teach them tools and give them resources on how to create meal plans, grocery lists, and easy-to-prepare, healthy recipes. I teach them portion sizes and what foods work best for their medical conditions. I teach them how to have sustained energy throughout the day and what foods increase inflammation. I look at their medical histories along with their food preferences and create plans. I give them honest feedback regarding their previous selections and we dialogue about any upcoming plans to their schedule involving food. I am their cheerleader, coach, teacher, and accountability partner all in one. I am one piece to helping them be successful.

The tools I provide are definitely valuable, but only one part of the process. One of the most important tools, and perhaps the biggest predictor of success, is the food journal.

The food journal doesn't lie. It tells you exactly how many calories you are consuming. It tells you if you didn't eat enough or ate too much for dinner last night. Sophisticated apps, such as Lose It! and MyFitnessPal, tell you how many macronutrients (carbs, proteins, and fats) and micronutrients (vitamins and minerals) each food you've selected contains. These apps can tell you when you've consumed too many milligrams of sodium or not enough calcium. They can provide you with immediate feedback on your selections—both good and bad.

I often tell my patients that in order to be successful, they must first exhibit awareness and ownership (accountability) before they can change. Journaling is an integral part of both. In the infancy phase, journaling can help you become aware of the type and volume of foods you are eating. Jour-

172

naling completely and honestly is taking ownership of your choices even when you don't want to reveal your shortcomings. Awareness and ownership always precede change.

When I first started my practice, I was a cash-only business. One afternoon, a potential new patient called to ask if I could help her lose weight. She proceeded to tell me that she knew everything there was to know about nutrition. She taught home economics (family consumer science if you are under the age of 30) and spent her day teaching kids how to meal prep, measure portions, and create balanced meals. Despite all of this knowledge, she found her own personal scale climbing and she couldn't figure out why.

"I really need help," she implored, "but, I don't think you can help me. Do you think you can help me?"

She went on and on about how she knows everything and didn't want to waste her money to hear information she already knew.

Yes, lady, I get it, you don't think I can do it. Young and fresh out of school, I started to doubt if I could help her. I didn't want her to come into my office and then not be able to deliver. I had visions of her becoming a disgruntled patient, leaving bad reviews online. Finally, I convinced her that I would do my best and asked her to fill out a three-day food record prior to coming in. Maybe a fresh pair of eyes would be able to identify the missing piece of the puzzle.

On the day of her appointment, I was so nervous. After getting to know each other a little bit, I asked to see her food record. She handed it over and what I saw next nearly shocked me to my core. Candy! The food log was filled with **candy**!

Remember, this is the same lady that went on and on about how she knew so much about nutrition during her phone consultation. I was thoroughly shocked and confused to find the volume of candy she consumed throughout the day.

Was she trying to trick me? Was she setting me up? No, that didn't make sense. She wouldn't pay me to trap me. Did she really not know anything about nutrition? Should she be in the education field? No, she seems intelligent; that wasn't it. What the heck was going on?

I didn't want to offend her but I also needed more information. I pushed the journal back to her and asked what she thought of her documentation. Her entire demeanor changed from our phone call of being aggressive and angry to humble and sincere.

"I had no idea," she sheepishly replied.

"Okay," I began. "Tell me more."

She proceeded to tell me how her coworker who shared a room with her had a candy jar on her desk. I don't remember the type of candy exactly, but I do remember it didn't require any unwrapping, so I'm going to go with gummy bears or something along that line. Every time she walked past her coworker's desk, she would grab a small handful of gummy bears, and every time she walked back to her desk, she would grab a handful more. This pattern happened every day, multiple times.

My patient also started to take notice that her coworker refilled the jar before leaving for the afternoon, making it hard to quantify how many gummy bears she consumed.

The most interesting piece was that the rest of this lady's diet was pretty much on point. She always ate a low-calorie, yet nutrient-dense breakfast, packed a salad every day for lunch, and cooked a balanced, nutritious meal for dinner. No wonder she was confused! The meals she sat down for and remembered eating were fantastic. It was the mindless eating that only a journal could pick up that was the culprit.

Since an extra 100 calories over and above one's needs can lead to 10 pounds in weight gain over the course of a year, it wasn't surprising why she was seeing the scale go up. I mean, 10 gummy bears are almost 100 calories (depressing, I know)!

We discussed tips for eating with intention versus mindless eating, and she figured out how to lose the unwanted pounds. Thankfully, I could help her, but not without the help of the journal. Had she not filled that out, she may not have remembered consuming them at all in a future conversation.

Journaling is the first step to becoming aware of your eating habits. It can be a powerful tool in helping you see patterns and quantity consumed. Whether you're a pen-and-paper type of person or tech savvy and enjoy using apps, what type of journal you choose to use isn't the most important decision. Reviewing and utilizing the data for future change is the key to the kingdom.

If you have never tried keeping a log, I challenge you to start, just for three days. Look for areas where you can improve your eating habits and start by choosing one habit to improve. Who knows? You may even find your own version of gummy bears hiding in there!

choose your plan

Affirmation

Repeat this statement every day this week:

"Awareness and ownership always precede change."

Action

The next time you order pizza (eat in or take out), also order a large salad to provide balance to the meal.

Achieve

For three days, calculate the grams of fiber you are consuming, either by looking at a food label or inputting your food intake into a food tracking system (I personally like MyFitnessPal). Average the three numbers and then slowly increase your fiber intake until you are at the goal (25 grams for women and 38 grams for men).

Analyze

Keep a food journal for three days and identify one habit you would like to improve as a result of your finding.

Accountability

Answer the below questions in your dedicated healthy lifestyle journal:

What change did you attempt to make this week?

Were you happy with the results?

What challenges did you encounter?

How would you do things differently next time?

5-star recipes

Banana Oat Pancakes

Pancakes rarely fill me up, but because of the added fiber, these stay with me all morning long. To make oat flour, simply put one and a half cups of oats in a food processor and process until they resemble the consistency of flour. Be sure to pay attention to steps five and six with timing since the consistency of these pancakes makes it hard to know when to flip.

Makes 6 servings

Ingredients

4 small bananas
1 tsp real maple syrup
1 tsp vanilla
2 eggs, beaten
1½ cup oat flour
2 tsp baking powder
½ tsp salt
½ tsp ground cinnamon
½ cup mini chocolate chips or toasted walnuts (optional)

Directions

1. In a small bowl, combine the mashed bananas, maple syrup and vanilla. Add the eggs and mix well.
2. In a medium bowl, stir together the oat flour, baking powder, salt, and cinnamon.
3. Pour the wet ingredients into the bowl of dry ingredients. Being careful not to over mix, stir the ingredients just until mixture is combined.
4. Let the batter sit for 10 minutes to thicken. Add chocolate chips or walnuts if using and stir to incorporate.
5. Pre-heat a nonstick pan over medium-low heat, or heat an electric griddle to 350°F. Once the surface of the pan is hot enough, pour ¼ cup of batter onto the pan. Let the pancake cook for about 3 minutes, until bubbles form around the edges of the cake.
6. Flip pancake with a spatula and cook for another 90 seconds until golden brown on both sides. Serve immediately.

Turkey and Black Bean Stuffed Peppers

Journaling full recipes versus individual foods can be difficult when using an app on your phone. Some of my patients get discouraged trying to type in each ingredient of a recipe due to the amount of time it takes to input the data. Although this method is the most accurate, it can eventually get very frustrating, leading to abandoning the practice of journaling altogether. If you've experienced the same aggravation, I urge you to simply enter the food item into the system and just pick the average calorie value. Remember, journaling is a system to bring awareness and ownership, which is far more valuable than precision and perfection. Speaking of time consuming, I used to make stuffed peppers by cutting off the stems and top portions of the peppers and then scooping out the inside. Who knew you could just cut the pepper down the middle? So much easier!

Makes 6 servings

Ingredients

Nonstick cooking spray
1 medium onion, chopped (about 1 cup)
1 tsp olive oil
1½ lbs. ground turkey
½ tsp ground cumin
¼ tsp chili powder
1 can (15 oz.) black beans, rinsed and drained
1 can (14.5 oz.) diced tomatoes
6 scallions, thinly sliced
6 medium bell peppers
1 cup shredded reduced fat Mexican cheese blend
1 cup salsa
¾ cup plain Greek yogurt
2 cups fresh cilantro, chopped

Directions

1. Grease a 9x13 glass baking dish with nonstick cooking spray. Preheat oven to 350°F.
2. In large skillet over medium heat, sauté onion in oil for about 5 minutes, or until translucent, stirring occasionally.

3. Add turkey, cumin, chili powder and cook until browned, approximately 5 to 7 minutes.

4. Stir in the beans and tomatoes with juice, and cook over medium heat, 5 to 7 minutes, stirring occasionally until mixture thickens. Stir in half the scallions.

5. Cut the peppers in half lengthwise and remove the seeds and membranes. Divide the turkey mixture evenly and spoon into bell pepper halves. Place the peppers in the prepared dish.

6. Top each pepper with cheese and bake 25 to 30 minutes.

7. To serve, top each pepper with salsa, yogurt, fresh cilantro and remaining scallions.

Source: Adapted from Tadych's Econofoods[2]

lesson 14

The Attention Your Body Deserves

"Your body can be your best friend or worst enemy.
It all depends on how you treat it."
—Unknown

We've spent some time building a strong foundation and developing strong layers along the way, because let's face it, we want to get it right this time. Treating your body properly means healthy self-talk, healthy foods, and healthy movement.

Choosing to make the right decisions all the time gets exhausting. We have to exercise our choice muscles like we do our regular muscles—with consistency, patience, and intention. Over time, the load gets easier to bear.

The following section walks us through the pains of making hard choices over and over as well as the beauty that follows. The words and actions we have repeated for so long become distant memories as they are replaced with new scripts.

Our bodies do an amazing job taking care of us each and every day. Imagine what we could accomplish if we treated them with love and respect. Imagine the energy we would have if we poured life into our bodies instead of poison. Imagine the impact we could have on others if we drew from a source of power and energy instead of constantly draining and depleting our resources. Our bodies are amazing vehicles wired for greatness. All we need to do is show them a little love along the way.

nourish

Valentine's Day Tradition

Five years ago, I told Jim the only thing I wanted from him on Valentine's Day was for him to cook me dinner and to clean up afterward. No gifts, no chocolates, no flowers, just dinner.

He enlisted help from the boys, researched recipes, grocery shopped, cooked, and cleaned up. The boys put up a curtain between the kitchen and dining room so the girls and I couldn't see what they were doing.

While the boys prepared dinner, the girls and I curled our hair, painted our nails, and put on fancy red dresses (read "fancy" as Christmas dresses).

Dinner was a four-course meal, including an appetizer, a salad, an entrée, and a dessert. The boys dressed up in ties to serve the meal and were so proud of their hard work. Afterwards, we turned on some music and spent the night dancing, switching partners so everyone had a chance to be involved. We all agreed it was the best Valentine's ever and declared this our new family tradition.

Every year the girls and I look forward to this holiday. The boys get into it as much as the girls. They try to outdo their performance from the previous year with more complicated recipes and indulgent ingredients. One year, Jim tried to beer-batter and fry cod. I was confused, because we don't eat a lot of fried food, so creating an oil bath to cook fish seemed a little lofty of a goal. When the fish exploded in the pot, it only added to the fond memories. I told him he could have made spaghetti and I would have been just as happy. Yet, I quickly learned that if you give the Delgado boys a challenge, they will rise to the occasion.

This Valentine's Day was no exception. The boys served us a cheese and cracker plate with French bread and homemade dipping sauce. For the entrée, they made tuna steaks served over lobster, homemade mashed potato cakes with a chive and bacon sauce, and a beautiful tomato salad. Dessert was a vanilla cake with icing and fresh berries, made from scratch by my oldest son. We danced before the meal, and in all honesty, I don't know if we could have moved after dinner from being so full. Our bellies were full, but so were our hearts. Valentine's Day is becoming my most favorite holiday, not because I don't have to cook or clean, but because of how much we all feel loved.

The Importance of Self-Love

Feeling loved is important. Feeling as if you belong is important. We are meant to live this life in community. We are meant to share in each other's joy, each other's burdens; each other's successes and each other's failures. "We" is always better than "me."

The idea of "me" is isolating. "Me" is fearful and has this amazing ability to invoke catastrophe into different situations. Just last month I broke down and told Jim I thought we were heading for divorce. He looked at me with wide eyes and bewilderment when I gave him the news.

"Where is this coming from?" he asked.

I told him we had a lot of conversations leading up to this in my head. He gently reminded me that next time I have these conversations in my head, he would like me to say them out loud so he could be an actual participant. This is why I love this guy so much. He sees my crazy and loves me anyway. Thankfully, my ability to overdramatize a situation such as this one is infrequent, and our commitment to marriage is stronger than any irrational thoughts that may pop up in my head from time to time.

"Me" also has the ability to think harsh words and create self-doubt. I used to think those harsh words would motivate me to try harder or shame me into doing better, but age and wisdom will no longer allow me to believe those lies. It is so important to monitor your self-talk, especially when it comes to your body. Your body is an amazing home to your organs and your soul. It takes a beat down from time to time, yet it continues to move forward.

If you find yourself talking negatively about your body (your stomach, your thighs, your butt), immediately replace the comment with a positive one.

"My stomach is so big and ugly," immediately gets replaced with, "My stomach was home to my babies."

"My legs are flabby," gets replaced with, "My legs are strong and carry me all day long."

You get the picture. Even if you don't believe it right away, say it anyway. Say it as many times as you need to until you start to believe it. Talk to yourself the way you would talk to your four-year-old self. You owe yourself that much. You owe your body love.

So what does showing your body love look like? It looks like rest when it is fatigued. It looks like movement when your body is restless. It looks like fuel when your body is depleted. It looks like warm baths and hugs when it feels unstable.

It also looks like kind words and positive thoughts. An amazing thing will happen when you start to give your body love. When your body feels loved, it will respond with kindness right back. It will supply you with energy and strength. It will give you a positive outlook. It will show you that you are more than capable of reaching your dreams.

Love is sometimes a choice. We are commanded in the Bible to love others as we love ourselves, but how does that work if we don't even love ourselves? Choose to love yourself today, tomorrow, and every day after that. Choose to do the work and then watch your body show you love right back.

eat

Stereotyping Cholesterol

Social media was in uproar when a photo was posted showcasing Trader Joe's newest milk product. The image revealed a milk shelf at the grocery store and a sign above it.

"Organic ... 2% MILK ... $5.49 ... VEGETARIAN FED CHICKENS ... 38% LESS FAT THAN WHOLE MILK ..."[1]

I'm not sure what you learned in school, but last time I checked, milk comes from cows (at least the stuff you buy in the store does).

This picture screams what is currently wrong with nutrition. There is so much confusing information out there and a lot of what you see is straight up wrong. This was quite obviously a simple mistake made by a clerk at the store, but wouldn't you be led to believe it in this day and age? Common sense is no longer our guiding principal and the need to bring it back is so important!

My goal every time I meet a new patient is to provide accurate information in a way that's easily digestible (pun intended). Anything less would be a disservice to my patients and a compromise to the level of excellence I hold myself to professionally.

Understanding blood work is an area of confusion for my patients. Sometimes they have had the opportunity to review their numbers with their doctors and other times they have pulled the information from a portal and are looking for help to figure it all out. In that case, I am able to use their results as a teaching moment.

Cholesterol confuses people the most in my experience. Most people know there is good and bad cholesterol (HDL and LDL, respectively), but they don't actually know the difference.

During the interview process for new patients, I ask if the new patient has any medical issues, such as high blood pressure, high cholesterol, or diabetes. Every now and again, I will get the joy of a chuckle when a person shakes his head and tells me he is perfect. Once we get to the medication section, I then find out the patient is on a statin. I gently remind him that statins are used for high cholesterol.

"But my cholesterol is fine," the patient will argue, without fail.

To that, I want to respond, "Yes! Because you are on a statin! The only reason it's fine is because the medication is making it that way."

For most of my patients, high cholesterol comes due to poor eating habits and inactivity. Every once in a while, it will be genetic. I tell those people their livers are overachievers and usually medication will keep it in check. We get cholesterol into our bodies in two ways: our liver makes it and we eat it in our daily diets. Interestingly enough, we now know that a diet high in saturated fat has more of an impact than dietary cholesterol.

The Working Chemistry of the Cholesterol Family

When it comes to fat, cholesterol, and reading lipid profiles, it can get a little confusing. I tend to improvise my explanations. Humor me, if you will, as I describe the following situation. **Warning:** I fully know I am stereotyping males and females. I'm okay with it. Please be okay with it too.

Let's pretend it's your three-year-old's birthday. Your three-year-old eats cake and ice cream. As a result, his hands are a sticky mess. Remember back to Jim's barbecue sauce nightmare ... what does a three-year-old do when he has sticky hands? That's right, he touches *everything*! The table, the chairs, the walls!

Now, a sticky wall could be wiped down, but what would be the fun in that?

"I can fix this," dad says, proceeding to break out his power sander to give the walls a smooth finish. He sands the walls and problem solved; except now there is dust and debris from the sander on the carpet.

No worries, mom is here for the rescue with her vacuum. All is well, because grandma was standing by with her vacuum too. The ratio of females to males has allowed for the crisis to be averted.

However, what happens if your three-year-old has his friends over? Now there are 14 kids running around your house touching the walls. Dad is doing his best to keep up with the kids, but he's outnumbered. He calls his brother, his neighbor, and all of his brother's neighbors to come over to help him out.

They immediately get to work, sanding walls, in an effort to stay on top of the kids. Mom and grandma are doing their best to keep up with the 15 men in the house, but they're falling behind. The ratio is off balance. The dads are trying to keep up with the kids and the moms are trying to keep up with the dads, but it's not working.

Think about your eating habits in this way. In this story, the kids represent poor dietary choices, such as high sugar and high saturated fats, which can cause inflammation. Studies show that increased amounts of either of these two nutrients are associated with higher LDL levels, higher triglyceride levels and lower HDL levels; all which point to higher cardiovascular risk.[2]

As long as HDL is in good ratio to LDL, our bodies can thrive. It's when the LDL rises, but the HDL stays the same (or decreases) that we have a problem.

We can talk LDL and HDL ratios all day long, but the more important question is how can we control the kids (which in this case represents inflammation)?

I have never been a fan of putting on Band-Aids when it comes to my professional career. I want to get to the sources of problems. There is no exception when it comes to cholesterol. Inflammation is caused by a number of things, including poor diet, lack of movement, smoking, alcohol, and stress. I have yet to meet a person who doesn't have a challenge with one or more of these areas.

In terms of food choices, selecting more plant-based oils over animal fats is a great way to keep LDL levels in check. Moving your body is a great way to increase HDL. It appears we're not getting away from diet and exercise any time soon. It is here to stay, because more often than not, it's the root cause of the problem. Abstaining from smoking, engaging in moderate alcohol intake, and practicing stress management are three other ways to manage inflammation.

A major strength of the human body is its resilience. It can take quite the beating before eventually wearing down. Even if you are currently on a statin, small changes can reap big rewards. One of my favorite parts of my job is working with patients and their physicians to decrease—if not eliminate—medications, while simultaneously creating a space for people to manage their ailments with diet and exercise.

I realize there are specific cases (re: overachieving livers) where an individual must stay on his or her medications, but that is not true for everyone.

What is one way you can improve your lipid profile right now? First and foremost, talk to your doctor about your health goals.

From a dietary standpoint, avoid trans fats and choose olive or avocado oil for cooking. Limit fatty and/or highly processed meats like sausage or salami. Engage in healthier preparation methods by steaming or baking instead of frying. Add fish to your diet twice per week for good heart healthy, omega-3 fatty acids, or add avocado to your sandwiches instead of mayonnaise. Choose more soluble fiber in the form of oats, oatmeal, beans, fruits, lentils, and vegetables. Add more plant-based meals into your weekly routine.

Walk around the block once or twice after a meal instead of sitting on your sofa to increase your HDL levels. Even if the changes feel small, it all counts. Everything you do makes a difference, so keep striving to live a healthier lifestyle.

repeat
Why I Run

I suppose I have always enjoyed running. In high school, I ran for the track team, mostly competing in sprinting events. I joined the team for one very important reason, because all of my friends were doing it.

I wasn't the fastest sprinter, but I could hold my own in the 100-meter and 200-meter sprints. In fact, when I was a junior, our 4x100-meter relay team competed in the state tournament, which was a big deal for a small farm school in Lancaster County.

My 4x400-meter team missed the qualifying time by hundredths of a second, but I can't say I was too upset about that race, because I hated that event. Four hundred meters is one time around the track. It was a difficult race, because it required sprinting for an extended period of time. There was no such thing as pacing yourself, because it was over in about a minute. You just needed to give it your all and hope you didn't hit the wall when you came off of that last turn on the track.

In college, after I put on a good deal of weight, I decided to go back to running. Because I was out of shape, once around the block was all I could handle. Over time, one block became two, and two eventually became ten. I built up my endurance one mile at a time until I could run for 30 minutes. Running could be lonely, so I passed the time by counting things. Doors, mailboxes, street signs, hills, songs on my Walkman (remember those?); whatever I could count, I did in order to pass the time. I enjoyed being outside and people watching. I also enjoyed pushing myself to accomplish new goals and distances.

185

I ran my first 5k while I was dating Jim. I had never even heard of a 5k before, but a couple of people from Jim's office registered for the race, so I decided to give it a try. Jim and I trained by running around his town. He was much faster, but didn't have great endurance. I was the opposite. Together, we pushed each other to achieve both. The two of us started placing at different races and I even ended up coming in first for women in one particular race. That was probably when my competitive drive set in and I started setting my sights on longer distances.

I ran the iconic Blue Cross Broad Street Run in May 2002. The race is a 10-miler down one of Philadelphia's most famous streets. It's flat and fast, which is great for building confidence. On the way home, I decided I wanted to run a marathon. I told my dad my goal. He laughed and then told me I was crazy. That was all I needed to hear. I was determined to prove him wrong.

My husband's boss at the time also wanted to run a marathon. He called me up one day and told me he signed up for the Pittsburgh Marathon. I couldn't understand why he would sign up for a race in one of the hilliest cities in the Northeast, but I also knew that if I didn't sign up with him, I might chicken out. My training began in January 2003. It just so happened Jim and I got engaged a month prior, so what better way to get in shape for a wedding than running a marathon? It made sense in my head, despite finishing up an internship and getting ready to sit for the dietitian exam. All I can say is I was a young overachiever. It makes me tired just thinking about trying to accomplish all of that at this stage of life.

I trained for five months following a beginner's marathon plan from Runner's World. I had no clue what I was doing, so I just stuck to the plan. If the training schedule said to run seven miles, I did it. If it said to rest, I rested. I also followed the "Run nine minutes, walk one minute" plan. This approach allowed me to run further and created the mental break I needed every 10 minutes. Once my mileage started to increase, Jim would meet me with water and snacks to refuel. We were a good team.

The race itself was definitely challenging. My goal was to just finish the race, but I secretly set out to finish in less than four hours. The Pittsburgh Marathon is known for being a difficult course. The last half of the race is all hills, with the most significant incline presenting around the 12th mile at Oakland Hill.

Luckily, the local hills did a great job preparing me for the race. My game plan was to run the race exactly as I trained, alternating nine minutes of running with one minute of walking. Once I started the race, I felt good, so I decided to go with it and just kept running. I ended up needing to stop and stretch at mile 20 and 22. Other than that, I felt like Forrest Gump!

Now, it wasn't all rainbows and unicorns. I was extremely close to making a costly mistake during the latter half of the race. Because a marathon is a long, 26.2 miles, it's important to fuel oneself throughout the race. Some runners choose carbohydrate beverages, while others consume snacks along the way. I chose GU, packs of carbohydrate-rich gel that were easy to digest and provided me with the necessary energy my body needed to continue on. It didn't taste that great, but it did the job.

At one water station, I saw volunteers handing out Popsicle sticks with what looked to be GU smeared at the end.

"Hmm ..." I wondered, "I should probably take one of these and eat it so I can save my own supply for later in the race if I need it."

Thankfully, I watched the man in front of me grab a stick and subsequently rub it on his nipples! It wasn't GU, it was Vaseline! Apparently, that distance can cause chaffing for men. Could you imagine if I had put Vaseline in my mouth? Ugh, the thought makes me ill!

I was elated when I finished the race in my goal of under four hours; however, after all the training and hard work, I needed a mental break. I didn't end up running again for an entire year. Soon after, I got pregnant and then pregnant again, and running became a thing only people who had time and energy did.

I started to realize why the 35-and-older bracket became the largest, most competitive bracket in races for females. It was filled with women who needed to get away!

Fifteen years later, I am running 15 to 20 miles per week, just for fun. I rarely do races, mostly because I'm competitive and don't want to lose. I also don't want to burn out, so I try to run with friends so I can talk and make the time go faster. I strategically try to ask my friend, Alyssa, thought-provoking questions before we climb a big hill to make her do all the talking, but she's on to me now.

I tell Jim all the time I enjoy the physical effects of running, but benefit more from the mental effects. Some people struggle to see this connection, but running provides an outlet to reduce stress. Running gives my anxiety and my worries a place to go out of my body and onto the sidewalk.

When we're stressed and overwhelmed, we have a feeling of needing to get that emotion out of our bodies. If we choose to eat during moments of uncomfortable emotions, we push those feelings back down into our bodies. Unfortunately, the reality is they are still there, wanting and needing to escape. From personal experience, I can assure you that they will come out one way or another, despite your attempts to push them back down. For some, that eruption will come out in the form of screaming. For others, it will come out through expanding midsections. For some furthermore, it will cause gastrointestinal distress.

Running, for me, creates an outlet for the emotions to leave. I remember our pastor talking about the Dead Sea and why it is such a nasty body of water. When you look at it on a map, the Jordan River flows into it, but there is nothing flowing out of it. There's no outlet, causing it to be one of world's saltiest bodies of water. Imagine how healthy the water supply would be if it had an outlet. Imagine how healthy your body would be if it had an outlet.

About six months ago, I had some routine blood work done, showing an elevated BUN and Creatinine, insinuating kidney problems. I didn't think much of it, because I had worked out prior to giving blood and figured I didn't hydrate properly. I got retested and the blood work was normal.

My doctor wasn't as blasé about the results and told me I needed to make sure I was prioritizing dealing with stress and hydration properly, because apparently my kidneys were showing signs of being affected.

Stress? In my life? I have five kids and own a business, yes, but I countered that I felt pretty good, despite having occasional stressful moments. She gave me a deep breathing worksheet and told me to practice the art every day.

I think that's why I gravitate toward running. Running forces me to pay attention to my breath. The rhythmic cadence of inhaling and exhaling mimics intentional, deep breathing. Even though I'm physically moving, the breathing part of running is relaxing, relieves stress, and is rejuvenating. It's why I run.

So, it makes sense why I tell my husband I need to go for a run for my mental sanity. It also makes sense why the most popular and competitive age group among women runners is 35–50. We need our outlet so we don't become salty.

The good news is you don't have to run marathons to achieve the same result. There is something extremely powerful when you combine fresh air, sunlight, and movement. That movement can come in the form of walking. Start by walking around the block. Over time you may find yourself having the endurance to walk 10 blocks or even attempt a 5k. After that, the possibilities are endless!

choose your plan

Affirmation

Replace negative self-talk with positive self-talk every time you catch yourself saying something unkind.

Action

Walk, jog, or run outdoors this week. Combine sunlight, fresh air, and movement for a powerful pick me up.

Achieve

Add avocados to your meal plan this week. The recipe for green hummus that follows is a good place to start! Bonus points for adding two servings of fish to this week's meal plan too.

Analyze

Show your body kindness this week by either taking a warm bath, feeding it a balanced meal (include the starch), and/or taking a 20-minute walk outside. Journal your mood and how your body felt afterward.

Accountability

Answer the below questions in your dedicated healthy lifestyle journal:

What change did you attempt to make this week?

Were you happy with the results?

What challenges did you encounter?

How would you do things differently next time?

5-star recipes

Spinach Avocado Hummus

I stumbled across this recipe preparing for a Girl Scout nutrition talk, and I doctored it up with added spices. This hummus is a great snack with pita chips or veggies, plus it's loaded with heart healthy, omega-3 fats, which we learned are great at reducing our LDL cholesterol.

Makes 8 servings

Ingredients

2 cups spinach
1 medium avocado
¼ cup Parmesan cheese, grated
2–4 cloves garlic
1 tsp salt
3 TBS lemon juice
4 TBS chives
¼–½ tsp red pepper flakes (optional)
2 (15 oz.) can garbanzo beans, rinsed and drained

Directions

1. In a food processor, puree the spinach until mostly smooth. Add avocado, Parmesan, garlic, salt, lemon juice, chives, and red pepper flakes. Continue to blend until combined and pureed.
2. Add the beans and pulse until well incorporated.
3. For best results, allow the flavors to marry in the refrigerator for 1 to 2 hours before serving.

Source: Adapted from Super Healthy Kids[3]

Basil Walnut Pesto

My boys do not disappoint on February 14, when it comes to creativity or culinary skills. This pesto is a great example of how they take normal chicken or fish to the next level (plus, it's more economical to use walnuts over pine nuts, which is the traditional ingredient in pesto).

Makes about 10 servings (1¼ cups)

Ingredients

2 cups gently packed, fresh basil leaves
2 large garlic cloves, roughly chopped
½ cup grated Parmesan
⅓ cup walnuts
½ tsp salt
¼ tsp ground black pepper
⅔ cup olive oil

Directions

1. Place the walnuts and garlic in a food processor fitted with steel blade. Coarsely chop for about 10 seconds.

2. Add the basil leaves, salt, and pepper and process until the mixture resembles a paste, about 1 minute.

3. With the processor running, slowly pour the olive oil through the feed tube and process until the pesto is thoroughly blended.

4. Add the Parmesan and process 1 minute more. To prevent the pesto from turning brown, you can store the pesto in a tightly sealed jar, covered with a thin layer of olive oil. Pesto will keep in the refrigerator for one week. If you're planning on freezing it, omit the cheese and stir in once you defrost it.

Source: Once Upon a Chef [4]

lesson 15

When Life Gets in the Way

"Your present circumstances don't determine where you can go;
they merely determine where you start."
—Nido Qubein

So, you've encountered your first hiccup. It's now time to see if you will sink or swim. Is your foundation strong enough? Will you make the right decision? The world awaits your next move.

You may have been making some great changes to your overall health, but there will be this one moment where the healthy choice becomes hard. It feels like your future success hinges on this one decision.

As much as I want Jim to know exactly what my needs are in every single moment, he is not a mind reader. For example, I was in the mood for ice cream when he was going out to pick up one of our sons from basketball practice. I asked him to stop at Sonic on the way home and pick up a small dish of ice cream for us to share later. Without stopping to take a breath, I quickly told him I didn't want it.

"Am I supposed to get it or not get it?" he asked, confused.

"You decide," I told him, knowing his question was valid.

I wanted it, but also didn't want it. I wanted him to make the right choice for me. Who doesn't want ice cream? Then again, who wants the extra calories?

In this section, we will tackle the confusing issues like phantom diagnoses, dining out, and figuring out what diet is best for you. Put your thinking cap on; it's a requirement for this lesson!

nourish

Selective Mutism

Although I love public speaking, I'm an introvert. My tendency to find the nearest wall in a room full of people is obvious proof. As a kid, I wouldn't even pick up the phone to order a pizza. I was too scared. My dad once threatened me with the choice of either making the phone call or the whole family not eating. I chose not to eat (and he eventually called it in—thank you, dad!).

I suppose I inherited introversion from my mom. Jim is on the quiet side, but has no problem approaching strangers and talking to them. I find it all fascinating.

My kids are on the quiet side too. Don't get me wrong, my boys are crazy in their own ways, but in large group settings, they tend to be more reserved. So, it was no surprise when the girls were on the shy side too. They never talked to strangers and went as far as turning their bodies away from people if anyone tried to start a conversation with them. We chalked it up to them being twins and always having a conversation partner. They chatted with the immediate family as well as our babysitter non-stop at home, so we didn't see it as a problem.

One Friday night, we were at a local community night and ran into some friends. My friend, Shannon, also happened to be the director at my kids' preschool. She bent down to talk to the girls to ask them if they were having fun that night, and they immediately put their heads down without responding.

I answered for them, as I had become accustomed to do, but Shannon interjected, suggesting a professional evaluation instead. I was defensive at first, explaining that my girls were fine and that they were just shy, but Shannon gently nudged me to think about it.

So what if they didn't talk *once* in preschool the year before? So what if they physically turned their bodies away from people when approached? How can this be a problem? It was the first time I started to think she was right.

The following year, when the girls entered the four-year-old's program at their preschool, we decided to separate them so they could start to prepare for kindergarten the following year. Bella was holding her own in her class, but Charley was struggling. She has the stubbornness of a bull and would not participate despite various attempts on her teacher's behalf.

My dear friend, Carrie, was Charley's teacher that year. She tried everything to get my little girl to open up on her own. Carrie was studying to become a school behavior therapist, so I knew God had put her in this position for a reason.

Carrie approached me about a diagnosis called selective mutism, which basically means the child chooses the people who she converses with. The reason we, as parents, were unaware of the condition was because the girls talked normally at home. Carrie continued to explain that if not nipped in the bud, the condition could affect the girls' ability to do well in school as so much of young children's assessments are done based on verbal feedback. If there was no feedback, it would be assumed the child did not know the answer and she might be labeled incorrectly as needing additional services. Enough said. I called the intermediate unit to sign them up for an assessment.

As we drove to the county unit, the girls started to question where we were going. I had no clue what to say, so I made it up on the spot. I told them we were going to go into a room where a teacher would ask them questions to see how smart they were.

They seemed to be fine with that answer and we proceeded into the room. Since I couldn't set two appointments in the same day, I had to do one girl on that day and come back for the other the next day.

Bella went first. The teacher asked her questions and she answered back! The girl *rarely* answered anyone, yet that day was the day she decided to open up.

The next day when they assessed Charley, the same thing happened! She had *never* talked to anyone outside of our family once in her entire life and that was the day she decided to talk.

The examiner took me aside to explain selective mutism, unaware of my previous knowledge of the condition. That was when I realized my girls were smarter than me! They completely knew what they were doing, and if challenged, would rise. Unbelievable!

The teacher walked them to the sticker room to pick out a sticker and they returned to their nonverbal states. Bella left without a sticker, crying the whole way home because she didn't pick one out. Charley at least pointed to the one she wanted.

Meanwhile, I tried to explain to the examiner that this was the behavior we were seeing in public. The examiner told me the testing portion was over and she couldn't use the new information on her assessment. The whole experience was absolutely mind blowing.

Believe it or not, the girls did not qualify for services because of their communication in the assessment room (big surprise). Instead, the examiners gave me a few resources for people who potentially could help, but didn't live anywhere close to my house.

I called Carrie to tell her the news. Her brilliance preceded her as she devised a sticker chart reward system for my girls! It was slow to start, but it worked like a charm. We created the same system for Bella in her classroom. Slowly but surely, the girls started responding and even raised their hands in class (seldom, yes, but they still did it!)

The girls are now in first grade and are each thriving in different classrooms. My elementary school is amazing. I tell Jim all of the time, we cannot move until all of the kids have passed through that school.

I met with the guidance counselor before the girls started kindergarten and she agreed to allow the girls to come into school before the year started in order to become acclimated to their environment and gain confidence. She personally assigned the girls to teachers she thought they would connect with and thrive. I'm happy to report both girls are doing extremely well and both their past and present teachers do not see any signs of selective mutism. It's amazing to see how much they have grown.

Speak Up!

Although many do not have a formal diagnosis like selective mutism, I often see patients who don't speak up for their needs.

My favorite clients are couples, because I get a glimpse into their lives and am reaffirmed of the normalness of my own marriage. Whenever I counsel couples, we always start with how to communicate needs to each other, especially if both are working on similar goals.

In the example of weight loss, I tell them they need to work together, to lean on each other's strengths, and to be supportive. I teach them how to truthfully communicate what is helpful and what is not. For example, if I tell Jim I need to pull back on my calories because we have been eating out too often or eating too many desserts, it is **not** helpful for him to question my choices by saying, "Are you going to eat that?" If he says that, then I am going to want to eat a double portion. I feel threatened and judged. Neither emotion ends in my favor. What does work for me is not asking me to go to Rita's for Italian ice, and instead, taking the kids on a night I work late; or, being enthusiastic when I tell him I want to go for a run. That is helpful.

In order to be successful, we need to be open and honest with each other. It's the only way. What conversations do you need to have with your spouse or significant other right now to help you be successful? One example may be, "I know you like to surprise me with my favorite snacks and I really appreciate it, but can you please not bring ice cream home at night? It's hard for me to say no, and I'm working hard not to eat after dinner. Recently, I've been eyeing up these new yogurt flavors at the grocery store I would love to try for breakfast. Instead of after dinner treats, maybe you could surprise me with them!"

Another response could be, "I love spending time with you and watching movies, but I have been working hard at finding ways to be more active. How about instead of our weekly Sunday matinee, we alternative movies with walks in the park?"

What conversations do you need to have with your coworkers or friends to help you stay on track? Be specific on what is and what is not helpful. For example, I had one patient who lost motivation whenever someone at work gave him a compliment on his weight loss successes. Instead of motivating him to keep working hard, he viewed it as the opposite and wanted to give up since other people were noticing, almost as if he'd reached his goal sooner than expected, so no need to keep going.

Even though other people noticing results may be helpful to some, it's not true for everyone. As a result, we brainstormed comments that would be motivating to him. He returned to work and told his coworkers, "Thank you so much for noticing my efforts; however, what would be even more encouraging is to ask how much water I've consumed today, or if I got to the gym this week." Once he gave them specific examples, they could help him stay on course. It's important to give others the exact sentences to either use or avoid, as people are not mind readers. Don't forget to ask others how you can help them be successful too! We're all on this journey together, so it's important we work together instead of expecting each other to know exactly what we need.

eat

Don't Forget to Wear a Lifejacket

These are the words I should have said to my 8-year-old son, Ben, before he went out in a boat with his oldest brother and dad … in the rain … during a flood warning: "Don't forget to wear a lifejacket!"

The rain was nonstop that weekend and the creek beside our house was rising. On our way to church, the boys asked if they could take the boat out, since they had never been in it before.

Mistake Number 1: Listening to a 12-year-old's logic. When I say boat, picture a small, canoe-like form of transportation with a 180-pound limit. My husband weighs 180 pounds. My oldest son, Jake, at the time, weighed a little more than 100 pounds. I'm guessing Ben weighed around 80 pounds.

Mistake Number 2: Doing the above math and still agreeing to let the boys on a boat over 100 pounds beyond its weight capacity.

Mistake Number 3: Since we only had one oar, Jim nonchalantly used a garden hoe to use as the second oar. (Please don't ask me how we lost the other oar. It's most likely in the black hole with everything else that is missing from our house.) That solution made perfect sense to me—find the garden tool with the least amount of surface area and use it to paddle your way down the stream. Apparently, the thought process was that they could use it to push off of rocks.

Mistake Number 4: Letting one of the kids use the hoe as his oar. Jake lost the gardening tool pretty much right at the beginning of the boys' excursion. If our garden is not thriving this summer because of our inability to move dirt, I will have no hesitation in reminding them of their costly mistake.

Mistake Number 5: Ignoring the set stopping points. The water was really fast. I get it—fast equates to fun and I'm sure they were having a blast. However, because the stream was moving so fast, the boys kept moving past the original stopping point (don't forget they only had one oar). "No problem," they thought, "we'll just keep going and find out where this leads us."

Mistake Number 6: Hitting a tree. According to Jim, this was going to be a good thing, because it was going to stop the boat and provide a landing spot to get out. Except when they hit the tree, Ben must have leaned over from the impact, bringing a ton of water into the boat and eventually capsizing it. Jim said the water was about waist high on him, which meant it was chest height or higher for Ben.

Mistake Number 7: Where was Ben's lifejacket? As Ben made his way to the bank, the current grabbed hold of him and he ended up going under the tree and coming out the other side. Thankfully, he grabbed on to two dead branches until Jim could get to him. The boys made it to safety and left the boat lodged next to the tree to hopefully recover the next day. They had a nice walk home, probably laughing the whole time about their adventure.

When they got home, Ben told me he didn't know if he was ever going to see me again and he wasn't being overdramatic; it was a pretty scary experience for an 8-year-old. The next morning while eating breakfast, Jim was singing "Survivor" by Destiny's Child to Ben. It must have gotten into his head, because I heard Ben humming it when he was getting his backpack together. Ben asked me if we as a family could celebrate his life every February 11, with pizza and ribs. I told him that could absolutely be arranged, as long as I could include a salad.

Strap on Your Lifejacket
Before Jumping into a New Diet

As I recounted the day's events to my friend, Carrie, we made jokes of the situation and how it was a good thing I wasn't there to witness what went down. Jim is an amazing father, but in this case, there were just one too many mistakes that could have resulted in an alternative ending.

Crucial Mistake Number 7, not wearing a lifejacket, gets us into trouble, both physically and metaphorically. From a nutrition standpoint, jumping into a new way of eating without creating a plan often leads to disastrous outcomes. Where I see this the most is when my patients dine out at a restaurant.

We go out to eat for a multitude of reasons: pleasure, community, but also for convenience. Oftentimes, when we are trying to eat healthy, restaurants present a difficult challenge, because we are forced to make hard decisions. Should we choose the salad or the cheeseburger and French fries? It's excruciatingly hard to pick the veggie and hummus plate when the words "wings" and "ribs" are listed right below it. We often treat restaurants like vacations, blowing off the health factor, because it's "an infrequent event." The problem is we aren't treating dining out as an infrequent event anymore. For most of my patients this is a four- or five-times-a-week occurrence between breakfast, lunch, and dinner. We are now at a point in time when people eat out more than they cook at home.

I had a patient once tell me the first time she ever stepped foot into a restaurant was on her 18th birthday. I realize that's a little extreme for this day and age, but it's a wakeup call to how often we are engaging in this convenient act. If we treat eating out like vacations, it won't be too long until our pants can't keep up with our expanding waistlines.

So, how do we navigate our way around this? The obvious answer would be to not eat out so often, but for some people, this is not an option. Many vocations revolve around entertaining with meals either once or twice a day. Since most people do not have the option of quitting their jobs, we have to figure out another way. Here are four tips to a successful restaurant experience:

1. **Aim for 500–600 calories per meal**—This piece of advice gives you

two alternatives: choose a meal in this calorie range or split a high-er-calorie meal into halves, thirds, or even quarters, to make your portion fit into this calorie range.

2. **Look at the menu ahead of time**—This is a big one! It's too difficult to make healthy decisions in the moment when you're faced with a bunch of unhealthy items on a menu. Add in some of the smells and sights from other patron's tables and it's a recipe for disaster. Choosing what to eat ahead of time from your home or office allows you to think clearly with your goals in mind. Once you decide what you want, do not look at the menu when you get to the restaurant—that is just a tease. Why would you do that to yourself? It's just mean!

3. **Order first**—Let's say you do decide to go with a healthier item, but then once you start to hear your dinner companions ordering more indulgent items, you change your mind. Ordering first lets you set the stage without being persuaded by others' decisions.

4. **After dinner, make sure you move!**—Walking after a meal is a great way to help digestion and decrease blood sugars. If you don't have time for a walk, at least park your car as far away from the restaurant as time permits. This tactic will help you get a few extra steps into your day and counter some of those additional calories from your meal.

repeat

'I Think You're Gluten Intolerant'

A few months ago, the perimeter surrounding my eyes was seemingly infected with an itchy, irritating rash. I was equally embarrassed by the sight of the red dots and afraid to use makeup to cover them up. I couldn't think of any recent changes I made to my makeup or food intake, so I was stumped on why they were rearing their ugly heads.

I happened to have my annual physical scheduled, so I brought it up to my doctor.

"I think you're gluten intolerant," she said, citing that any rash around the eyes usually had a strong link to a gluten allergy.

She recommended I remove gluten and dairy from my diet for three weeks. At week four, I was to reintroduce dairy, followed by gluten at week six.

Desperate to clear up my face, I obliged and got straight to work on meal planning. The girls' birthday was right around the corner, so I found a gluten-free, dairy-free cupcake recipe, because if mom has to change, everyone has to change.

I followed the diet to the letter for three weeks and nothing changed. My face looked just as red and irritated as ever, despite completely changing my diet per the doctor's orders. To say I was irritated by the lack of results might be an understatement.

Next, I mentioned the issue to my gynecologist at my annual appointment, embarking on a mission to get all of my doctor appointments in around the same time and taking full advantage of asking the expert opinion of anyone I could find with a medical degree.

I asked her if she had ever heard of a rash around the eye being tied to gluten sensitivity and she looked at me like I had three heads. She mentioned her friend was sensitive to parabens and that I should buy paraben-free makeup, face wash, and shampoo.

To me, tossing all of my makeup from high school and buying new, expensive products seemed a little excessive if I wasn't sure it was definitely the cause. After all, I had been wearing makeup sporadically for years and never once had an issue. I had a hard time believing a paraben allergy would just appear out of thin air.

I decided to do my own experiment and discontinue wearing makeup as well as any makeup remover in favor of my already paraben-free face wash.

The rash started to go away after a few weeks, and after adding my makeup back to my routine, the rash still didn't come back. The new makeup remover I purchased a few months prior—despite being gentle, sensitive, and paraben-free—must have contained an ingredient that caused the allergy. My near-three-month experience of living with the embarrassing rash finally came to an end.

Dr. Google Told Me I'm Gluten Intolerant

Thanks to the recent popularity of the Paleo and Whole 30 diets, most people inaccurately assume they are gluten intolerant and start asking questions about how they can eliminate the villain from their diets. I agree some diagnoses fare better at eliminating the protein gluten from the diet, but it most certainly is not an absolute for everyone.

Eliminating gluten is not easy and certainly not glamorous. This lifestyle change is difficult and should only be followed if absolutely necessary. Our jobs as dietitians are to educate, not to scare people into following the latest fad diet. I have no ill feelings toward the doctor who gave me the wrong information. I think she legitimately felt like it was the right course of action.

As a result, I found some great gluten-free, dairy-free recipes for my patients to use who actually have intolerance.

We have so much information at our fingertips through Google, WebMD, and social media, we are sometimes at a disadvantage. Self-diagnosis is rarely a good idea. We all know too well the dangers of Googling a dry cough. Pretty much every Google search can lead you to your ultimate death.

There is nothing wrong with trying new foods to experiment with feeling your best. Trying new things leads to knowledge—either you found something new that works or found an option that doesn't. Either way, you still have more knowledge than before.

One benefit to all this information is a network of people ready to share their experiences and provide insights on what was helpful to them. I often read message boards with people experiencing rare conditions for guidance on trusted resources to research.

Whenever you do research on the internet, The National Institute of Health tells us to keep five things in mind[1]:

1. Who created, runs, or moderates the site or app? Is it a trustworthy individual or source?
2. What is the site or app promising or offering? Do its claims seem too good to be true?
3. When was its information written or reviewed? Is it up to date?
4. From where was the information derived? Is it based on scientific research?
5. Why does the site or app exist? Is it selling something?

Learning how to research wisely and effectively on the internet is an important tool to have in your back pocket. It might possibly have saved me a month or two of aggravation in my own journey.

choose your plan

Affirmation

Repeat this statement every day this week:

"It's up to me to ask for help.
Other people cannot read my mind."

Action

Choose one or more of the four tips discussed in "Eat" the next time you dine out.

Achieve

Next time you seek medical advice from Dr. Google, use the guidelines outlined by the National Institute of Health to help you navigate your research on the internet. Always talk to your doctor before you take action.

Analyze

What conversation do you need to have with your family member, coworker, friend, or neighbor to keep you on the right track with your health goals? This week, commit to having that conversation. Bonus points if you return the favor by asking how you can help that person stay on track with his or her goals!

Accountability

Answer the below questions in your dedicated healthy lifestyle journal:

What change did you attempt to make this week?

Were you happy with the results?

What challenges did you encounter?

How would you do things differently next time?

5-star recipes

Tart Spinach Salad

This is my usual, go-to salad when I'm looking for a side dish to bring to a potluck. Bringing a salad ensures you always have a healthy choice over all other options. Making your own salad dressing may seem daunting, but this one couldn't be easier!

Makes 4 servings

Ingredients

For the Salad
> 10 oz. spinach
> ½ cup dried cranberries
> 1 medium Granny Smith apple, chopped
> ½ cup walnuts (or pecans), chopped
> 2 oz. goat cheese, crumbled

For the Dressing
> 3 TBS olive oil
> 1½ TBS apple cider vinegar
> 1 TBS Dijon mustard
> 1 clove garlic, minced
> 1½ tsp honey
> Salt and pepper, to taste

Directions

1. In large bowl, combine spinach, cranberries, apple, walnuts (or pecans). Top with goat cheese.
2. In a mason jar (or container with lid), combine salad dressing ingredients and shake to combine. Serve with salad.

Almond-Crusted Chicken

This dish is a gluten-free alternative to fried chicken. Since it is baked and not fried, it is a much lighter version to the greasy original.

Makes 4 servings

Ingredients

For the Chicken
- 1½ cups almonds
- 2 eggs, beaten
- 4 boneless, skinless chicken breasts
- 1 TBS olive oil

For the Spice Mixture
- ½ tsp dried sage
- ½ tsp dried rosemary
- 1 tsp dried thyme
- 1 tsp dried oregano
- ¾ tsp onion powder
- ¾ tsp garlic powder
- 1½ tsp sea salt
- ½ tsp black pepper

Directions

1. Preheat the oven to 350°F. Place a cooling rack on top of a baking sheet.
2. Place the almonds along with all the ingredients in the spice mixture into a food processer. Pulse until almonds are ground. Transfer to a bowl.
3. In another bowl, add the beaten eggs.
4. Dip the chicken in the egg, then coat in the almond spice mixture. Lay each piece on the baking rack.
5. Drizzle the olive oil over the chicken and bake for 45 minutes until golden brown.

lesson 16

Know Thyself

"Ask yourself if what you're doing today
is getting you closer to where you want to be tomorrow."
—Unknown

Just like a waitress checks on her patron's food, it's time to do a little self-evaluation about the changes you have made up until this point. Are the changes taking you closer to or further away from the end goal?

Self-reflection is an integral part of the process. It allows us to celebrate the things that work and identify the current challenges that still exist. If we delude ourselves and never course correct from time to time, we may one day find ourselves very far from our destination.

One of my patients was recently met with a question from a friend, "What is your secret to your weight loss?"

Since she's been successful in her efforts, she answered, "It's actually really easy. I eat lots of fruits and veggies, I exercise, I stopped drinking a lot on the weekends, I drink a ton of water, and I get a lot of sleep at night. Oh, and I see a dietitian for accountability every month to make sure I keep doing all of those things."

Whether we need accountability or the guidance of a trusted professional, check-ins are what keep us on the path to success. Experience and muscle memory will guide us, but there will always be new circumstances to navigate. Introducing the practice of self-evaluation from time to time ensures the straying is kept to a minimum.

nourish

Life Lessons from CVS

About a year ago, I took the girls with me to CVS to pick up a prescription for one of the boys. The antibiotic wasn't quite ready when we arrived, so we proceeded to wait in the back of the store next to the pharmacy. There was a small magazine rack located under the pharmacy counter, and right smack dab in the middle of the rack, that month's issue of *Women's Health Magazine* was prominently on display. It just so happened Sofia Vergara was on the cover that month, strategically sitting on a stool, accompanied by the caption, "Strong Sexy Naked," in big, bold, italic letters.

Since the magazine was exactly eye level with my then-five-year-old girls' line of vision, they were immediately drawn to the picture.

"Mom, why doesn't that lady have any clothes on?" one of them asked.

"I'm sorry, honey, what did you say?" I replied, half listening. My eyes were drawn to where they were pointing. "Wait, why **doesn't** she have any clothes on?"

I immediately shielded Bella and Charley from sight of the magazine, but the damage had already been done. They had made a beeline for it, flooding me now with questions. The girls were on a mission to find out everything they could about this risqué photo.

"Does she know someone took a picture of her without clothes on?"

"I'm guessing she did since she covered her privates, but this was not a good choice," I replied.

"Is it okay to let someone take a picture of you without clothes on?"

I grew both angry and sad. Angry that my five-year-old daughters were subjected to this visual in what was supposed to be an innocent trip to the drug store; sad that my kids were asking these types of questions.

"No!" I fired back. "It is *never, ever, ever* okay for someone to take pictures of you without your clothes on!"

I was in shock. I felt completely unprepared, yet still I searched the depths of my mind for a way in which I could help create a teachable moment for my girls. I frantically spouted out the first thought that popped into my head.

"Mommy is going to turn all of these magazines backward on the shelf," I said. "I know if I didn't have my clothes on, I wouldn't want people looking at me, so let's give this lady the same respect. If we turn them around, other people can't see her either."

Both girls were happy to help, because that's something five-year-olds are very enthusiastic about. As we started to pick up the magazines, one of the girls began to ask more questions.

"Is she fat?"

"Wait, what?" I doubled back. "What did you say?"

"Is she fat?"

"Where is this coming from?"

"Look at the girl in that other picture," she said, pointing to the Sports Illustrated conveniently placed next to Women's Health, showing a different woman, wearing a sports bra. "Are they fat?"

"They are not fat," I responded. "Why would you even ask that question? Honey, neither of these women are fat. You know what? Let's turn these magazines over too."

After we turned all of the magazines over, I was reminded of an article I read about a father of a seven-year-old girl who took a side-by-side picture of the magazine covers of Girls Life and Boys Life. Both magazines were targeted towards preteens, but had very different messages. The Girls Life magazine featured stories, such as, "Wake up Pretty," and, "Your Dream Hair," while the Boys Life magazine posted headlines reading, "Explore Your Future," and, "Stories of Scouts in Action." The message was clearly different for girls and boys and that is unacceptable.[1]

Growing up is hard enough without having magazines give you messages that you're not enough unless you look a certain way. In the case of Women's Health Magazine, why couldn't Sofia Vergara just be strong and sexy with her clothes on? I get it … to sell magazines and ultimately make more money, but at what cost?

My colleague, Molly, told me she no longer reads women's health and beauty magazines to avoid the emotional roller coaster. She explained that you first open the magazines excited from the headlines on the front covers. You feel encouraged reading the editors' notes, but then quickly become envious of all the products you don't own, but feel like you should, so you can look like a model.

You start to feel motivated by the exercise sections, directing you to look like the thin models in the pictures, but the next page will tell you to love your body the way it was created and to celebrate what makes you different. The next page may feature a chocolate-frosted brownie, which implores you to treat yourself to a cheat day. The repetitive highs and lows you experience are just too much. I had never thought about it that way before, but I couldn't agree more.

So, what's the answer to all this? Clearly, I can't visit every CVS across the nation, turning magazines over to help shield the eyes of innocent five-year-olds. As much as I was annoyed at CVS for putting this magazine at my kids' eye levels, eventually (after a long time), I was thankful for the dialogue it opened up between the girls and me, knowing full well this would certainly not be our last conversation about the topic.

Every day, I tell them that they are the most beautiful in their hearts and if they aren't beautiful in their hearts, it won't matter what they look like on the outside. I teach them their worth doesn't come from size, but how they treat others. I teach them that people make poor choices and we need to all help each other out from time to time and build each other up. It's easy to teach these lessons to five-year-olds, but harder to believe them at age 38, after years of society conditioning us otherwise. Personally, I choose to keep trying until I get it right!

Thank you, CVS, for life lessons for us all.

eat

Stupid Swedish Fish

It was Fourth of July and our family upheld its annual tradition of attending the Skippack Community Parade. My two oldest boys typically drive to the parade with my mother-in-law two hours before the event to get a good seat and save our spot now that close to 35 of us attend—a gathering of aunts, uncles, cousins, and close friends that have built up for more than a decade. It's a tradition that we have come to look forward to every year.

Guilty pleasure time: my absolute, most favorite candy in the world is the red Swedish Fish. I don't need anything flashy—no sour warheads, sticky airheads, or chocolaty tootsie rolls—just simple red Swedish Fish. Since this Fourth of July parade throws out candy, historically it has become typical for one of my kids to catch one of the snack-size bags of sugary goodness. I have made it clear to each one of my kids that if anyone should be lucky enough to catch one to politely toss it my way. I don't ask much from them. Thankfully, all of them agree and don't give me too much of a hard time at my request.

What I didn't realize was that this particular year the good people of the Skippack parade must have nominated Swedish Fish as the official candy of 2018. After roughly 20 floats passed by us, I had seven bags of Swedish Fish on my lap. When Charley threw me her first bag, I happily ripped it open and ate the five pieces of red deliciousness. But then, Jake, Ben, and Bella threw me their bags, and shortly after, I got another bag from Parker. I was so excited and thrown off by the sheer magnitude of Swedish Fish bags that I just started ripping bags open and eating the contents.

It didn't take too many more floats passing out the candy to get a stomachache, so I told the kids to save the rest of the bags for themselves. Thank goodness I don't have quite the same affection for other candy and was able to call it quits after my initial sugar rush.

After the parade, we made plans to go to our local pool to swim since it was so hot outside. Jim and the boys wanted to watch a special on the history channel first, so I sat on the sofa to join them. Not too much later, I felt my eyelids get heavy, and within minutes, I was snuggled on the sofa enjoying a nice, afternoon slumber.

I woke up confused and not quite sure where I was or what time of day it was. Did I just take a nap? I don't even remember the last time I took a nap. Was it 2011 when the girls were babies? I don't take naps. This was so out of the ordinary for me! I started to replay the day's events to see if I could figure it out.

Maybe it was my workout that morning. It was leg day and I was in the third week of a new strength-training program. I didn't think the workout was that strenuous, but maybe it was harder than I thought. I started to feel a little bit of pride well up in my chest. Was I that much in shape that I couldn't tell the difference between a hard and easy workout?

Or, maybe it was the heat. We did just sit outside in the hot sun for the past hour and a half. Except, we really didn't. We were under a beautifully shaded tree, which made the parade quite comfortable. Was it warmer than I had judged it to be? Had the heat exhausted me? Did I not drink enough water?

Then it hit me. The pride that puffed my chest immediately deflated. It was those stupid Swedish Fish! I was coming off of a sugar rush and crashing. The nap was a reaction to eating too much sugar in one sitting!

Curiosity: Nature's Original Mode of Education

There is a lesson we can all learn from this: always become curious about how you feel. If you're responding "oddly' (in this case it was my need for a nap), ask yourself why. I knew deep down that the exercise and heat weren't the real causes of my fatigue, even though I wanted to believe they were. Becoming curious about the situation is what finally led me to the real cause.

I had a client who recently told me his button popped off his pants and his immediate thought was, "Maybe I put my pants in the dryer too long and now they are shrinking." The scale on the other hand, confirmed he had gained five pounds.

The same can apply to you. If you're struggling to stay awake in the middle of the afternoon when you are at work, ask yourself why. Did you not get enough sleep last night? Did you eat a heavier lunch? Have you been sitting in one position too long? Becoming curious will help you determine outcomes of behaviors and give you feedback on whether or not you want to continue those behaviors.

Even deeper than this is a lesson on progress. I sincerely feel like choosing to eat nutritious foods works in this way. It's not a light switch that you turn on and off. You're not going to eat poorly one day and then magically make all the right decisions the next day, never having to worry about struggling again. I started to beat myself up a little bit about the Swedish Fish fiasco once I figured out they were the cause. Then I started thinking about the last time I overate candy in general. It took me a few moments to realize the last time I overate any candy was probably around Christmastime. That was a seven-month gap. I can live with that.

That's how progress is made. You may be looking to change a habit of your own. As much as you want to turn that habit off and never worry about it again, it doesn't work that way. So, you make a few changes, but there may be a little bit of regression from time to time. Soon, the length of time between committing your old habit starts to lengthen. You may only overeat candy twice a week. Over time, twice a week turns into twice a month, and before you know it, it's been seven months.

Be sure to give yourself some grace from time to time, because progress doesn't happen overnight. If Swedish Fish reign as the official parade candy once again next year, I'll be ready. However, I'm secretly hoping they nominate another type just to make it a little easier on me.

repeat
Consistency Over Perfection

I don't know how many times I have heard, "I used to be able to eat anything I wanted and not gain weight."

I find that my patients who struggle the most are former athletes (think: high school and collegiate days, not professionals). Most athletes create poor eating habits, because they have both a teenager's metabolism and hours of exercise logged in to offset the damage.

Your trusty dietitian, author, and (I hope) mentor is just as guilty of this, dating back to her teenage years. I grew up in a small town and went to a small school, graduating with under 200 fellow students. I was able to play multiple sports, since the school was small, and made the team of whatever sport I set out to play. I was fairly athletic and could hold my own on tennis courts, soccer and softball fields, and the track. I won several trophies and competed at the district and state levels. There were times I even played two different sports in one season.

Although I was having the time of my life, I was also picking up some really bad eating habits. I was learning how to slam down an entire meal in less than four minutes, because I was rushing from one practice to the next. Since I was burning so many calories, I didn't see how the taco buffet bar at Wendy's or the large Blizzards from Dairy Queen after a track meet were setting me up for challenges later in life.

What these people and my younger self chose to overlook is the continuation of old eating habits in a more sedentary environment, such as sitting at a desk from 9 a.m. to 5 p.m., never fares well. An individual's body is simply not the same at 40 as it was at 18, especially with less exercise.

Another reason former athletes struggle is they forget their bodies are not young and flexible anymore, making them more prone to injury. They push themselves and have expectations of playing at the level they enjoyed when they left the sport 20 years ago. They forget to stretch, or choose not to, because of lack of time. They experience plantar fasciitis or arthritis in their knees from years of abuse. Rather than warming their arms up slowly, they tear their shoulders after pitching to their kids on a Sunday afternoon.

I made the same mistake playing tennis last year with a patient. I was serving and hitting overheads like I never left the sport. Without fail, I ended up injuring my shoulder and I was shut down from exercising for a while. Not smart at all.

All or Nothing Gets Us Nowhere

I find this a lot with exercise. We're either going to the gym six days a week or not going at all. It's rare to find the healthy in-between. Yet another reason former athletes struggle is the mindset around the structure and definition of a workout. High school and collegiate athletes train two to three hours per day while in season. Training is intense, and some sports require a second practice later in the day.

My former athletes have a mindset that in order to get a good exercise session they must sweat their butts off for at least an hour; otherwise, throw it out the window, because it doesn't count. I found myself victim to that same mindset, not working out at all because I couldn't find a window to work out longer than 20 minutes due to other responsibilities. I needed at least an hour for it to count because that is how I defined exercise. So, another day would go by without movement or exercise ... and another ... and another ... until months went by and I was getting more and more frustrated by my lack of progress.

My light bulb moment came when I realized 20 minutes was always better than zero minutes. In 20 minutes, I could get a reasonable workout in and feel good about crossing it off my to-do list. The most important part was I could be consistent with the new workout routine. I wasn't killing myself, which meant I wasn't causing injuries. I slowly built up my stamina and time, and have continued my exercise regimen for the past five years. Yet, it started with just 20 minutes.

I once heard we should never exercise for weight loss. Exercise is for heart health, stress management, and better sleep; not for weight management. This is for two reasons:

1. What happens when you meet your goal? You don't have to exercise anymore? Of course not!
2. If you only associate exercise with weight loss, you may come to resent it and eventually quit. I find this to be true with many patients. I can't tell you how many times I've heard, "I should exercise more, and then maybe I'll lose weight faster." You might, but what happens if it doesn't work that way? Does that mean you stop exercising? Of course not!

When you constantly connect exercise and weight loss, the results are never long lasting. It becomes a conditional activity. It's only when you view exercise for the health benefits it provides that you create a habit for life.

The Fitbit exploded in popularity a few years ago, because it gave us insight into how sedentary we had become. I had patients tell me they would pace up and down the hallways at 11 p.m. just to reach the magical 10,000-step goal.

I was so excited to buy one, but my husband didn't share in my enthusiasm.

"Why do you need a watch to tell you to move more? Shouldn't you just move more?"

I wanted to see the numbers, so I bought one for my birthday with some gift cards, and it worked … at first.

I volunteered to water the garden to squeeze in some extra steps, since our garden is far away from our house and we have to carry watering pots back and forth to water the plants. I joined challenges and pushed myself to do a little better each week.

Over time, though, I started to tire from all of that pushing. I realized I was becoming resentful of the Fitbit and felt like a failure when I didn't reach a goal or win a challenge. I was even having moments where I wanted to stop exercising altogether, because it was becoming too much.

I decided to stop wearing the fitbit and reminded myself of all the reasons I started exercising in the first place. Remember, if an action step you are taking is moving you further away from your goal, it's time to readjust!

How do you view exercise? How are you exercising right now? How often do you change up your routine? Are you currently moving your body in a purposeful way? What changes could you make right now to improve your outlook on exercise?

I challenge you to start moving today if you aren't currently doing anything purposeful. Start with just a walk. Start with 20 minutes. Bring along a friend or family member and begin to change your life.

As with any health habit worth adopting, consistency always trumps perfection. Set out to be consistent in your workouts and see the amazing benefits of exercise!

choose your plan

Affirmation

Repeat this statement every day this week:

"Consistency trumps perfection, every time."

Action

Move your body in a purposeful way for 20 minutes for a minimum of three times this week. Choose exercises such as walking, jogging, biking or yoga. Bonus points if you exercise outside.

Achieve

Take a moment and evaluate the areas you go to for advice on health and beauty, such as magazines or the internet. Are these resources making you feel better or worse about yourself? Identify sources that aren't leaving you feeling encouraged and unsubscribe.

Analyze

Identify one habit you have changed over the past year. What action did you take to make yourself successful? How can you apply that same technique with a habit with which you are currently struggling?

Accountability

Answer the below questions in your dedicated healthy lifestyle journal:

What change did you attempt to make this week?

Were you happy with the results?

What challenges did you encounter?

How would you do things differently next time?

5-star recipes

Jimbo Special

Looking for a healthier version of a banana split? Yes please! Jim made this concoction one morning for breakfast when we were on vacation in South Carolina. He yelled to the kids, "Who wants a Jimbo special?" The name stuck, and to this day, it is still how I name the recipe when I share it with my patients. This recipe is a great breakfast, post-workout snack, or whenever you need a boost of energy.

Makes 14 servings

Ingredients

¾ cup low-fat cottage cheese
3–4 large strawberries, sliced
2 TBS crushed pineapple in its own juice
½ banana, sliced
1 TBS peanut butter
2 TBS granola
Drizzle honey (optional)

Directions

Combine all ingredients in a bowl and enjoy!

Yogurt Kisses

This quick and easy snack will feel like a special treat, but is really high in calcium and protein, so it won't put you into a sugar coma like Swedish Fish did to me. I like to eat these as an after-dinner "dessert."

Makes 1 to 2 servings

Ingredients

1 single-serve container of flavored Greek yogurt

Directions

1. Spoon the entire contents of the yogurt container into a Ziplock bag and seal.
2. Cut the tip off of one corner and turn it into a piping bag.
3. Pipe the yogurt into Hershey kiss shapes onto a sheet pan.
4. When finished, allow to set in the freezer for about 1 hour before enjoying.

lesson 17

Nurturing and Growth

"Change is inevitable. Growth is optional."
—John C. Maxwell

Growth is exciting. My kids are so excited when they grow taller or need the next shoe size. My oldest son is now officially taller than me, his handbreadth and shoe size have already surpassed that of my own. It's exciting to see him become a young man. It's also a little sad knowing my little boy is not so little anymore.

When it comes to our garden, we spend weeks preparing the soil, pulling the weeds, and hilling up dirt for planting. That part of gardening is not fun. On the other hand, walking out to the garden each day and seeing progress from the day before is exciting. Yes, you heard me right—watching produce grow is exciting. Have you ever seen asparagus grow from the ground? If the weather is warm and sunny, you can literally see inches of growth in one day! If I ever get to the point in my life where I have nothing to do, my goal is to sit outside and watch asparagus grow.

Watching my patients grow in both knowledge and experience is super exciting too. Walking with them in this journey is fulfilling on so many levels. My heart often feels like it's going to burst! It's exactly how I feel watching my own children accomplish hard things.

Change is hard, but growth is exciting. We're putting on the final touches and watching something beautiful evolve. Once we figure out how change works and our purpose is defined, we are empowered to do more—to continue growing and impacting more lives. My hope is that we never stop learning and growing.

nourish

Unworthiness

I find that I'm constantly struggling with my position as a dietitian and a business owner. Do I teach people what they want to hear (eat less, lose weight, look like a model) or teach them what they need to hear (you are worthy, you are beautiful, and you are amazing just as you are)? The former gets paying customers in the door while the latter shows love, compassion, and truth. Is there room for both? I wasn't sure.

Upon reading Oprah's book, *What I Know for Sure*, I came across a chapter containing a conversation between Oprah and her trainer, Bob Greene. They were in the middle of writing the book, *Make the Connection*, when she realized she needed a reminder about what the connection actually was. Bob taught her that her overeating was not about the food but the feelings behind the food. He repeatedly told Oprah that her weight was connected to her feelings of unworthiness.[1]

In all honesty, I skimmed over that section of the book without a second thought. However, when I arrived at the next page, the weight of those words sunk in.

"Hold up!" I thought. "What did I just read?"

I reread the passage.

"I totally disagree with this," I said, this time aloud in an empty room. "Who does he think he is for making a blanket statement like this?"

I continued reading the rest of that chapter internally declaring my opinions as truth and Greene's as fallacy. Yet, for some odd reason, this sentence would come back to periodically haunt me over the following few days. It was as if a seed was planted that afternoon that just needed time to grow and cultivate.

I had some internal investigative work to conduct. I had a yearning desire to figure out why that statement was bothering me so much.

I called and enlisted the help of my friend, Carrie. As a behavior therapist, Carrie has the uncanny ability of processing my thoughts. She is a great listener (even when I ramble) and is thoughtful with her words. She's a highly skilled therapist, because she always validates my thoughts by carefully rephrasing my dialogue. I always feel heard and safe.

"This is a fascinating revelation for you," she reassured. "What parts of the sentence are hitting close to home for you?"

I rambled in circles, but it eventually became clear to both of us my position on the matter.

I have never felt good enough.

I struggle with self-esteem. If I think back to my childhood (I hate those phony shows that make you go back to a time in your childhood, but here I was), I have always struggled with feeling good enough. In elementary school, I desperately wanted to be in the gifted program, but never was tested, despite my straight-A report card and finishing my work before anyone else. Inside, I was screaming, "Notice me" but no one did, so I worked harder.

In high school and early college, almost every single boyfriend cheated on me. Every boy, but one. I tried harder, compromised my personality, and tried to become the person they wanted me to be, but ultimately always fell short.

When I met Jim, he was 10 years older than me. I felt intimidated and inferior in the early goings and struggled to find my place in his world. He never asked me to be anything I wasn't, but I felt an immense pressure to not screw this relationship up, as well. Since he was older, I equated wisdom with age and compromised my needs and ambitions to meet my perceived role. I saw the people he gravitated toward and I was the opposite.

He worked next to a hair salon where most of the girls dressed cute, hair perfect, waxed bodies, and nails groomed to perfection. I was a t-shirt and mesh shorts kind of girl with my hair usually in a ponytail. I wasn't as thin as the other girls and secretly berated myself for not trying hard enough.

Why couldn't I get this part of my life under control like the rest of my life? I vowed to work harder. I was skeptical of any female relationship he had, constantly seeing others as a threat. It was a dark place that wasn't healthy for me or for us as a couple.

I carried those insecurities with me for at least a decade. Every so often they creep back into my psyche but the frequency has definitely decreased over the years. I'm not sure if that's maturity or wisdom, or maybe a little of both.

Now I'm reading a passage that links weight to feelings of unworthiness and I'm starting to connect the dots. For so long, I battled the feelings of "not good enough" as a thorn in my side. I tried to justify my own feelings of inadequacy with the thought, "struggling with my own weight and not feeling good enough is what makes me a good dietitian," and "this is how I can connect to my patients."

More dangerously, I thought God wasn't allowing me to look the way I thought I should, so I could show empathy and create a real connection with my patients. Twisted, I know, but this is my uncensored vulnerability at its finest. The reality is, God is after my heart.

The truth in all of this is I was already worthy just by being born. I am enough not because of what I accomplish, but because I'm a child of God. He chose me and loves me more than any human can! When He created me, he not only chose to love me, but also hand-picked special gifts and talents, which He wanted me to share with the world. How amazing is that? I can derive confidence from that and that alone. I don't need a six-pack or perfect hair and nails to win God's approval (or Jim's).

My purpose in life is not to achieve the perfect body, but to help others in their journeys, freeing them from the lies they were fed by ads and society. My purpose is to teach confidence in treating the body with love and kindness. My purpose even extends to teaching others they are enough just as they are and that Jesus declared each person's worth when He died on the cross. Well, how about that? Maybe Bob Greene was onto something after all.

eat

The Clean Plate Club

Do you belong to the clean plate club? I totally am a card-carrying, full-fledged member. I, like many children of the Baby Boomers, was taught to finish my plate before getting up from the table. I was told I couldn't have more of my favorite foods until I finished the vegetable. I was also told I couldn't have dessert unless I ate my entire dinner.

The image of my brother pouring applesauce sloppily all over his green beans is still embedded in my brain after all these years. His method was intended to make the green beans go down easier. To this day, I gag thinking about my experience of smelling and tasting sauerkraut every New Year's Day. We were forced to take down two forkfuls of the stringy, pungent cabbage if we wanted to proceed with the rest of our meals.

My parents are not evil people. They were teaching my brother and I to not be wasteful, just like their parents taught them. My grandparents grew up in the age of the depression, so it makes sense they were hyperaware of food waste, drilling the same ideals into the young minds of their offspring.

Food waste is a terrible thing. According to a 2012 report from the National Resources Defense Council (NRDC) the following statistics show you just how big of a problem it is[2]:
- Americans throw away $165 billion of food each year.

- 40 percent of food is wasted in the U.S. every year.
- 35 million tons of food are wasted in the U.S. each year.
- The average American household throws away $2,200 of food each year.
- The average American throws away 300 lbs. of food per year.
- 20 percent of food the average American buys is never eaten.
- 90 percent of food is thrown away too soon. Food waste in America has grown by 204 percent since 1960 and 50 percent since 1990.
- Reducing food waste by just 15 percent would be enough to feed more than 25 million Americans every year.

As a society, we are in desperate need of making a change. We can start by looking at the reasons food waste is a problem. The NRDC cites lack of education, lack of meal planning, creating shopping lists that do not provide accurate estimates of the food a person actually needs to buy, unnecessary impulse and bulk purchases, and over-preparation as contributing factors. We live in a time when large portions have become the norm, but this can lead to uneaten leftovers that end up being thrown away.

"The food on your plate will always go to waste—either your waistline or your waste can, so choose wisely." This statement, which I frequently say to my patients, is meant to be funny, but it sends the wrong message. The problem at its core (for a First World country) is excess. We take more food than we need *and* we overeat.

Physical plate sizes, in general, have increased over the past 60 years too, from 9 to 11 inches or more. It's not rocket science; larger plates allow for more food.

We visited Syracuse a few years ago to attend a former coworker's 40th birthday celebration. The party was held at an award-winning restaurant. When they called us up to go through the buffet lines, there were no plates … only platters!

Jim and I looked at each other as the person in front of me grabbed his serving platter and proceeded to walk through the line. It was hard to quantify how much food to take, because there was so much white space.

After consuming a quarter of my plate, I started to feel full. My gut reaction was, "This can't be right, I'm not anywhere close to being done." Thankfully, my brain reminded me I wasn't eating off of a normal plate. Imagine being part of the clean plate club at a restaurant that serves you platter-sized portions. You and I both know it wouldn't end well.

Bypass Guilt and Shame by
Listening to Your Body

Being a part of the clean plate club may help reduce waste, but it does nothing for physical or mental health. Overeating past fullness can lead to feelings of guilt or shame. It does for me, that's for sure.

We attended the wedding of one of Jim's relatives and were seated with his cousin, Lisa, who is in fabulous shape. We were all enjoying our meals and talking when Lisa, with a natural flow, pushed her plate slightly toward the middle of the table and announced she was full.

Analyzing her plate, I noticed half a dinner roll, a forkful of green beans, and about two bites of chicken remained. "You've got to be kidding me," I silently judged. "Is she seriously not going to finish the four bites left on her plate?"

Then it hit me! She stopped when she was full. She listened to her body instead of eating past fullness. It didn't matter if she had three bites or ¾ of the plate left. She stopped when her body told her it was time to put the fork down. This was a huge realization for me.

I once read, "If you want to be thin, mimic thin people—do what they do." I only knew how to be a clean plate member. I didn't know any other way.

Full transparency, I'm still not the best at leaving food on my plate. I have taken steps to decrease my portions, but my husband leads the charge on this one. We only eat off of smaller, salad-sized plates at home, and if we go out to eat, we almost always share meals.

Having a large family does help minimize overeating, because when you make an 8x8-inch pan of brownies for a treat and cut them into nine squares, there's only enough for one per person. We almost always eat leftovers for lunch. Ever since we started buying the veggie tray, our food waste has decreased substantially. Gone are the days in which we buy volumes of produce and throw pounds of spoiled product away, because we were too lazy to cut it up. Plus, even if it does start to look questionable, I quickly roast it for dinner that night.

The farm wields benefits for our family as well, since we can give our chickens any unwanted scraps or compost our produce.

I'm learning that it is okay to be part of the clean plate club if you're eating appropriate portions and listening to your body. The message here is that awareness is key. It's the first step to making change.

Eventually, the goal is to minimize excess food in totality—both in consumption (your waistline) and in refuse (your waste can). What is one practical way you can reduce food waste right now in your own household? If you are a member of the clean plate club, what one change can you make to meet your health goals?

repeat

It's Never Too Late

I was 38 when I officially learned how to apply makeup. I was 38 when I first started washing my face at night too. Now, it's not that I hate makeup ... I just never really figured it out before. You're really never too old to learn how to master a new task.

I was in Home Goods recently, and my girls asked me why the lady that just walked by was so fancy. She wasn't dressed fancy by my personal judgment, but her hair and makeup were done. Their follow-up question was, "Why are you never fancy?"

Ouch!

The truth of it all is, I don't like washing my face at night. I don't like waiting for the water to warm up, so most times, I would use cold water in my impatience and end up waking myself up instead of winding down. Further, what I really hate about washing my face is when the cold water runs down my arms as I'm trying to rinse off the soap. I hate that feeling, especially if my sleeves happen to fall down in the process. Now, not only am I awake, but I have wet, cold sleeves.

Logic says that if I don't want to wash my face at night, I shouldn't make it dirty; hence, no makeup. Although my friend, Carrie, argues I should wash my face for the simple fact that I existed that day. I think that's being dramatic, but what do I know?

I am fortunate to have found some great friends in the last decade. We make it a priority to meet for breakfast one Saturday morning per month. We rotate restaurants (or houses), and arrive promptly at 7 a.m., which is a miracle in and of itself, because Sara is not a morning person.

One evening, to celebrate Carrie's birthday, we decided to go out for dinner, but first met at Ulta. For those of you who have visited an Ulta, you know why it was completely overwhelming for a girl like me who didn't wear makeup. I get that same feeling when I walk into a craft store; more on that in a moment.

Carrie and Sara were at home as soon as they walked through the automatic doors of the beauty emporium, speaking in a foreign language I could not understand. I was able to make out a few words—contouring, eyelid primers, moisturizing creams—but did not interject. Eventually, our friend, Crystal, joined the group and we found a sweet lady to help us figure out colors and products. I even got in on the action and tried on different concealers. We had fun looking for different items, and I left with a chubby lip pencil (that's what she called it) and some blush. I bought more makeup that night than I had in the past three years.

My interest piqued, my friends recommended I watch YouTube videos to get started. I found a video in which a lady with similar hair and eye color to me was the demonstrator, grabbed a notebook and pen, and took myself to makeup school.

I texted my friends and told them I finally figured out why I didn't like makeup. Makeup is a form of art, and one form of art is craft. Makeup is craft! I don't do crafts!

My first C was in art. Give me a science or math problem any day, but please don't ask me to draw a simple earthworm. I will stay up with the kids all night figuring out chemistry or KenKen, but building a person out of a two-liter bottle must go to their father. If it resembles a craft, I'm out.

Taking my freshly jotted notes on makeup into the bathroom, I made an attempt to find the right "equipment" to utilize for what I had just learned. Luckily, I had never thrown out any of the makeup I bought over the past 20 years, because it's barely used.

I found all sorts of different shades of powders. I don't own a moisturizer, so I used my husband's daily sunscreen as a base (thank you Jimmy D). I personally do not care for foundation, so I skipped this step. I then used concealer like war paint under my eyes, down my nose, across my forehead, and on my chin. Don't ask me why I chose those particular places—it was what the girl did in the video. For all I knew, she had some acne there and was trying to cover it up. This was no time to question her motives. If she did it, I did it too.

Next, I moved on to powder in order to set the concealer. I found shades of powder that I thought could double as contouring colors and I made fish faces to get just the right spot.

Smiling to get proper placement, I applied my blush, and then completed the process with a light powder to highlight. I must have been in hibernation for months to purchase that color!

The eyes were next in line, so I practiced layering colors and blending. Starting with small circles, I then moved to a wiper motion.

"It's actually all coming together," I thought.

I finished the look with mascara and my chubby pencil, now ready to face the world ... except it was 10:30 at night, so I settled for facing Jim.

Now, Jim isn't a fan of lots of makeup. He's a massage therapist and when ladies get up from the table, he hates to see the face cradle protector covered in makeup. Deep down, maybe that's why I never pursued it. I knew he didn't care for the overly made up look, so it was just easier not to be fancy (as my girls called it). I went downstairs and casually sat next to him on the sofa.

He looked over at me but didn't say much. A few minutes later he asked if I was wearing makeup.

"Do you like it?" I eagerly asked.

"It looks like you care," he nonchalantly replied back.

Jim's way of complimenting me sometimes comes out rude and I don't feel as though I was overdramatizing this situation. I burst into tears, assuming he thought I didn't care about my appearance until that point.

Trying to apply ointment to the fresh wounds he just created, he told me he meant that it looked as though I wasn't trying too hard, just the right amount of effort.

I stormed out of the room to wash my face, determined to get it right.

"Tomorrow is church and I'm going to nail this makeup thing to show my friends," my inner dialogue continued. "I will be fancy!"

The next morning was Justice Day at my church, which meant they highlighted a social injustice going on in the world and our community. The topic of focus was foster care. I cried so much during the service, as I watched the video of kids in need, and the more I tried not to cry to save my makeup, the more the tears came. Mental note: go back to Ulta and buy waterproof mascara.

Six weeks later, I was finally feeling as if I was starting to get the makeup routine down. I didn't even need to follow my notes anymore. I had memorized all of the steps! This is just one example proving that you are never too old to make a change.

Ignore That Annoying Voice

Change is funny that way. When you're ready to make the change, the steps come fairly easy. When someone tries to tell you to change, there is usually resistance. The same holds true to dieting. I can tell right away if someone is going to be successful or not. She takes ownership of the current situation, is eager to learn, and figures out how to stop making excuses. That combination of attributes usually indicates to me that she is ready.

Some of my most successful clients are in their 50s and 60s. I recently had a 61-year-old lose 75 pounds. She worked at a dessert factory and had access to free dessert once per week. Years of partaking led to serious weight gain and her doctor told her she was on the road to diabetes. Some might think 61 is too old to start worrying about weight loss, but it was the perfect time for this particular patient. She even hated to cook and was on a tight budget, so we created a plan using only canned products. We figured it out!

What is something that you have always wanted to try, but are listening to that annoying voice in your head that tells you not to, because you're too old, too young, too overweight, or too busy? Maybe you have always wanted to run a race, try rock climbing, take cooking classes, learn a new language, or (sigh) how to make a craft. Whatever the case may be, your current situation, especially age, should never be a factor in learning something new. You might surprise yourself and find it opens up the doors to more exciting opportunities. Choose to ignore the inner voice that says you can't and explore your fancy new world!

choose your plan

Affirmation

Repeat this statement every day this week:

"I am worthy for the simple reason that I was born."

Action

Sit for five minutes in prayer or meditation every day this week, absorbing the idea that your worth comes from being born versus your accomplishments.

Achieve

Identify one thing or action you have always wanted to try and then take the next step at turning it into a reality. For example, if you want to try a fun dance class, research online facilities near you, and then pick up the phone to reserve your spot. Write down your idea and action plan in your journal.

Analyze

List all the ways you will eliminate food waste this week in your journal.

Accountability

Answer the below questions in your dedicated healthy lifestyle journal:

What change did you attempt to make this week?

Were you happy with the results?

What challenges did you encounter?

How would you do things differently next time?

5-star recipes
Zucchini Stacks

My grocery bill goes down dramatically in the summer months, because we are always eating out of the garden. We tend to let our zucchinis grow to the size of small whiffle ball bats, and it can be tough figuring out what to make besides 8,000 loaves of zucchini bread to pass along as gifts. This recipe is great on its own or sandwiched between a sourdough roll.

Makes 6 to 8 servings

Ingredients

1 large (or 3–4 small) zucchini, sliced into ¼" rounds
1 bottle Italian dressing
1 jar roasted red peppers, drained
Large fresh mozzarella ball, sliced
1–2 cups spinach
1 small red onion, sliced (optional)
1–2 cups fresh basil leaves
Balsamic dressing (see Salad Bar recipe in Lesson 3)

Directions

1. In large bowl, marinate zucchini in Italian dressing. Place in refrigerator for 2 to 3 hours, or leave out on counter for ½ hour.
2. Grill zucchini over medium-low heat until zucchini is caramelized (browned on both sides), about 8 to 10 minutes per side. The key is to go low and slow so they don't burn.
3. Remove from grill and stack additional ingredients on top. Drizzle with balsamic vinaigrette.

Shrimp Tacos

Some magazines will tell you the way to looking younger is special creams or injections. Some will go as far as recommending plastic surgery options. When Taco Tuesday needs a facelift, look to this alternative to shake things up. This recipe is super easy to make when you need a quick meal on the table. My kids love the variation.

Makes 4 servings

Ingredients

> 1 TBS olive oil
> ½ tsp. crushed red pepper
> 24 peeled and deveined large shrimp
> 1 large avocado
> 4 limes, juiced
> 1 cup chopped cilantro
> Salt and pepper to taste
> 2 cups broccoli slaw (alternatively, use cabbage slaw)
> 8 corn or flour tortillas, warmed in the oven
> 2 mangos, diced

Directions

1. In nonstick skillet, heat oil and crushed red pepper over medium heat. Add shrimp and sauté for 2 to 3 minutes, or until opaque.
2. Mash together the avocado, lime juice, and cilantro. Season with salt and pepper.
3. Divide the shrimp, broccoli slaw, and avocado dressing between the tortillas. Top with mango and serve.

lesson 18

You Are the Master of Your Body

"If you listen to your body when it whispers,
you won't have to hear it scream."
—Adapted from a Cherokee Proverb

If you've learned nothing else from this book, I want you to understand this very important concept: you, and you alone, are the master of your own body. No matter what idea popular or trendy diets try to sell you, there is no one-size-fits-all ideal to follow. You are unique, you are special, and God has handpicked you for a specific purpose by giving you a combination of gifts and talents.

Your unique health journey means you are the best decision maker when it comes to your body. I can try to steer you in a direction that has worked for others and/or myself, but ultimately, you are in charge.

You get to pick which health goals to make. You get to choose what exercises to do. You get to decide how best to utilize your gifts. Take the time to listen to your body and it will tell you exactly what it needs. The key is sitting still long enough to listen without getting distracted by the noise of the world.

My personal method of teaching is through storytelling. With these upcoming final thoughts in mind, it's now time to add chapters to your own personal story.

nourish

Parker's Gift

It may be instinctual, but it's a blessing, nonetheless. I first noticed it when my second son, Parker, was younger, watching him interact with other kids. He was extremely empathetic and compassionate, even as a young boy. One of my earliest memories of catching him in the act of using his gift was when he was playing a game with his brothers. On the other side of the room, one of the twins rose from the ground, legs wobbling, to make an attempt to walk across the room. She crashed hard, and as if he knew it was coming seconds before it occurred, Parker was first on the scene to comfort her.

"Wow, he got up before I did," I thought. Even more impressive was his nonchalance. It was of no inconvenience to him.

Teachers and other moms have made similar observations of Parker's behavior at school. He has always been the first one willing to help others and has consistently shown kindness to everyone around him.

A classmate of Parker's was struggling to transition to middle school, but since he was in one of her classes, Parker helped her successfully make the shift and find her way.

In sports, Parker is always the first one to find the person struggling the most and give him suggestions for improving his game with words of encouragement. When he was in elementary school, Jim had the opportunity to eat lunch with him on his birthday. Jim was surprised to see Parker not sitting with all his friends from baseball, instead opting to change things up with a rag tag bunch of people from all backgrounds.

Parker has never been concerned with status or popularity. His gift is to see people's hearts, not their shells. I tear up thinking about it, because I know this is a gift to me too.

I have a gift too, by the way. My gift is making any situation about me. Your mother-in-law is driving you nuts? I can turn that situation into a story about how my kids drove me nuts this afternoon. Struggling to find time to work out? I can tell you stories for days about how I time manage priorities. Of course, I'm being a little sarcastic, but sadly I'm not being dishonest.

This is my biggest curse, both personally and professionally. Every day, I have patients coming into the office to see me for tools and strategies to make healthier choices. I realize the last thing they want to hear about is what is going on with me, so I sit on my hands and bite my lip to keep from talking.

I admit I am thoughtful, but I'm aware I need to remind myself repeatedly that the visit is about the patient and not me. I want to change so it becomes more instinctual, but it's work! It does not come naturally and is definitely not my actual gift.

What I'm learning as I mature, which is a plodding process, is that my ability to help others is limited if I'm so preoccupied with myself. If I rush to finish a sentence for someone, I miss out on the information he or she wanted to relay. When my patient simply agrees with the words I choose, we both miss out on an opportunity of growth.

If I make assumptions about his or her motivation based on our conversation without asking directly, I miss out on key pieces of information that is helpful in setting the patient up for success. When I send my professional representative to the appointment—the authority figure I want to portray because of my pride—I actually perform a disservice to my patients.

Every December, I write goals for myself and divide them into four categories: spiritual, professional, personal, and physical. The only goal to show up in more than one category is, "talk less and keep your mouth shut more." Again, it's a work in progress.

Despite my gift of gab, I know I'm exactly where I am meant to be professionally. God has enlisted me to help others, and hopefully, directly or indirectly bring them closer to Him in some way. I invite you to use your gift to help others too.

Your gift is that part of you that comes effortlessly—it's just who you are without trying. Parker doesn't have to try to be empathetic or encouraging, it just comes naturally to him. Life is hard—even harder without others to lean on and learn from. God gave all of us a unique talent and gift that's reflective of His character. We are tasked with using that gift to help those around us. How are you using the gifts God gave you?

Is your gift clear to you? If not, ask the people around you to help you identify it. Someone else may more easily recognize your unique qualities, so don't waste too much time by trying to figure it out on your own.

Unfortunately, we sometimes let our self-centered representatives interfere with the great works God has set on our hearts to perform. We need the people in our lives to serve as reminders of our purpose. That's the beauty of becoming—we're unfinished work, but we can choose to walk toward it just a little bit more each day. Thank you, Parker, for teaching and inspiring me to become more.

eat

'I Only Eat Organic'

Do you know anyone who claims they "only eat organic"? I'm sorry if you are actually the culprit, but to me, it can be a bit annoying. Now, before I get too far into this, let me take a moment and clarify there are certain people who need to eat organic for specific health reasons. I'm working with a patient right now who has a propylene glycol allergy, which is listed under natural and artificial flavorings; so, in order to ensure she doesn't get sick, she must choose organic foods only. This is **not** who I'm talking about.

I'm talking about those who say these words with an air of superiority, as if "organic" makes someone of an elite class. I have so many patients who walk into my office, going on and on about how they only eat organic produce, only choose organic meats, or only choose grass-fed, free-range, chicken that is on a daily massage schedule and hand fed bugs by a certified licensed feeder (okay, maybe that last comment wasn't true, but you get the point).

Let's talk about eating organic, going Paleo, being on Whole 30, or whatever diet you've decided to try this week or this season. Your diet is your personal choice and there's nothing wrong with your decision. If you find it works, you are happy with the results, and you can maintain it for the rest of your life, go for it!

In terms of weight loss, I tell my patients all the time, there are more than 100 different ways to lose weight—we just have to find the one that works for you. This usually takes a little bit of trial and error, but eventually, we get there and settle into a nice routine that produces results.

Problems arise when we start trying to force our ways onto others. It's one thing to be excited about what we are doing and offering advice when we are asked, but we open a big can of worms when we make others feel bad for not choosing our ways.

Talk to the Hand that Feeds You

Now, I think organic is great. Nobody wants to eat foods with a bunch of chemicals and pesticides, so if you have the funds to purchase only these products then by all means, choose that route. If you don't, that's okay too. There are other ways of taking a more organic path without overly breaking the bank. You could try starting a small garden if you have the space (or container gardens if you don't). Alternatively, you could opt to purchase from small, roadside stands or farmer's markets. Often, these farmers follow organic practices, but never pay the fee to have someone come out and certify them. Talk to the hand that feeds you so you can make the best decision.

I recently came across an article posted in the *Journal of the Academy of Nutrition and Dietetics* about a new program for dietetic interns, called the Nourish Program, created by the University of Texas. To summarize, this adjunct program will provide hands-on experience to dietetic students on gardening and cooking, in addition to the standard clinical, community, and management rotations. With the recent popularity of "farm to table," it has become clear that dietitians are entering the workforce with an expectation of teaching this lifestyle, yet they lack the skillset to both communicate and execute the practices. As a result, home gardening and cooking with home-grown produce are now introduced as part of the curriculum to meet the need.[1]

When I first read this article, I was beyond excited. This is right in my wheelhouse! This is what I live and breathe every day at our farm—the place we call home. How exciting to hear educational institutions are going to teach others what I feel is such a foundational principle and cornerstone to good health.

Believe me, there are so many benefits to gardening. Working outside in the dirt can boost serotonin levels, which can mimic the properties of antidepressants. Not only do gut friendly bacteria that live in the soil help the brain produce more serotonin, but I also find the rhythmic practice of weeding to be calming and soothing, yet productive.[2]

Physical labor, as we know, is great exercise. Plus, the nutrition benefits of eating foods right out of your own backyard instead of eating foods shipped across the continent means access to more vitamins and minerals in every bite. The thought of prospective dietitians learning this skill in college means more people will have access to the information and hopefully be able to make positive changes. Everyone wins!

Then, another thought crept into my mind, but mostly my heart. This is actually sad. The fact that we have to teach people in school how to grow and cook a carrot means we have become far removed from basic gardening and cooking skills. It wasn't too long ago that most people had a garden in their backyard (or at least knew where to find one). Now, we live in an era where most people eat foods out of a box.

I spend most of my day educating people how to include more produce into their diets. It's not a hard concept to understand, but extremely difficult to execute given our busy schedules and lack of resources. We have literally made it so easy to have access to fake foods that seeking out produce is considered a novelty.

When did farm to table become a thing? Fifty years ago, my grandparents would laugh out loud if you told them of this absurdity. Farm to table isn't a trendy way to eat; it's the only way to eat. How did we arrive at this grim fate? Who decided it was a good idea to trade health for convenience? The simple task of learning how to make a basic stock from root vegetables is not a trend, but a way to act as a good steward of our resources.

I am beyond grateful for the leaders of our education system recognizing the need to bring back such a foundational principle. For the past 10 years, I have been teaching preschool children how to eat the colors of the rainbow by bringing in a basket of produce and teaching them the names of different fruits and vegetables. It never ceases to amaze me how many children have absolutely no clue about the names of common produce.

I implore you, talk to your kids about where they get their food. Teach them basic gardening skills. If you don't have all of the knowledge, borrow a book from the local library. Support your local farms and show your kids how food is grown. Make farm to table **the way** instead of a trendy fad diet.

Organic Doesn't Always Equate to Healthy

I would be remiss if I didn't mention that organic isn't the catchall answer to following a healthy diet. You still need to read food labels. Choosing organic cookies or organic juices filled with tons of added sugars does not make you healthy. I have repeatedly seen patients who consume organic junk food, arguing they are healthy even though they consume more sugar than their non-organic counterparts. The word "organic" does not automatically give you a free pass to eat whatever you'd like, so choose wisely.

One of my patients was struggling with irritable bowel syndrome and the uncomfortable symptoms that go along with it. When we reviewed her diet, there were very specific foods triggering her symptoms. When I reviewed which foods they were, she was confused, because she was currently purchasing those foods in their organic forms. Her assumption was that just because those foods were organic, they were healthy and her body would be able to properly digest them.

I frequently have to remind my patients even though a food may be considered healthy by mainstream's standards, it may not be healthy for the individual. Ask any person with colitis and he will explain that fresh, raw vegetables tend to tear up his insides if he is currently experiencing a flare. Purchasing organic, raw broccoli will not make that person feel any better.

It's also good to note the word "natural" means nothing. There is no legal definition of the word when it comes to the food industry. Governing bodies frequently try to define the word natural, but end up arguing in circles and tabling the discussion for a later time. Just because your product says "natural" and has a picture of a barn on the front does not mean it came from a farm or resembles anything created in nature. Learning how to read a food label is one of the best investments you can make in your health and is truly the only way to make an informed decision (refer to Lesson 12 if you need a refresher).

repeat
Jillian or Bob?

If you are over the age of 30, you may remember the hit TV show, *The Biggest Loser*. Contestants competed for the opportunity to win $250,000 as a result of losing the most weight compared to other competitors. They endured fitness and nutrition challenges, met with various doctors and psychologists, and weighed in on an oversized scale every week. Most of us watched these episodes while eating a bowl of ice cream.

In the earliest seasons, there were two trainers. Bob was portrayed as the sweet man who was always everyone's cheerleader. Jillian was more of a hardcore, scream-in-your-face kind of trainer. People typically gravitated toward one style over another based on what they thought would motivate them the most.

I always thought it would be interesting to be on the show to see what happened behind closed doors. I think I would have picked Jillian as my trainer if given the choice, because she scared me and I wouldn't have wanted to disappoint her. I always said the people that ended up getting voted off first were the ones that would be the most successful, because they had to figure out how to lose the weight without the luxury of living on the ranch. They had to go back to jobs, families, and responsibilities, as well as find the time to work out.

The ranch was safe, but it didn't provide the contestants with any real-life obstacles. I guess that's why we never saw any reunion shows. The winners of the show may have ended up losing their weight-loss battles in the long run.

Most people think if they lived in the perfect environment, they would be successful too. It would most likely increase their chances, but it wouldn't be a guarantee. Look at celebrities. Here are individuals with indispensable incomes who can afford trainers, chefs, and dietitians 100 times over, yet still some struggle with weight. Maybe the perfect environment is not the answer after all.

In order to be successful, we have to put ourselves in a position to be successful. One of my favorite ways to illustrate this point is when Oprah Winfrey interviewed Kirstie Alley on her show. Alley battled her own weight issues for years and told viewers her personal story. When she was motivated to lose the weight, she moved all of her dining room furniture into her basement and moved gym equipment into the empty space. Every time she walked through the dining room, which was several times a day, she was reminded to exercise her body. After she lost her weight, she reported getting cocky and returning the gym equipment downstairs. Out of sight soon became out of mind and the pounds found their way back. Alley was motivated again to lose the weight, so she went back to habits that worked best for her. The gym equipment found a new residence in the dining room yet again.

Know Yourself—The Good and Bad

I'm a big fan of creating a plan and setting my patients up for success. Identifying potential barriers ahead of time allows them to work out the kinks so they don't become a distraction and eventual derailment. It's also important that we each take the time to review our strengths and our weaknesses.

For instance, if you are not a morning person, do not set a goal to wake up at 5 a.m. to exercise. It won't happen. If you don't like exercising by yourself, do not buy home-study programs. You won't do them. If you don't like waking up early, make your breakfast the night before. If you don't like cooking during the week, prep on the weekends. There is no one size fits all way to live a healthy lifestyle. You must lean into your strengths in order to create success.

One of my closest friends, Crystal, recently became a spin instructor, because she is motivated by being around others and she is extremely dependable. She wanted to work out more often, but was struggling to commit to exercise at home. She utilized her strengths by finding an exercise routine that worked for her. Knowing clients are expecting her to show up, combined with how much she enjoys working out with others, led her to the path of fitness instructor. If it's important, you will find a way. If it's not, you will find an excuse.

Find Your Way

I once had a patient tell me that exercise is like physics, quoting, "a body in motion will stay in motion and a body at rest stays at rest." If you currently exercise on a regular basis, you will resonate with this statement. If you currently do not exercise at all, you will also resonate with this statement.

The every-once-in-a-while exerciser struggles the most, because it takes so much effort to get started. There is a strong inertia to overcome. Finding momentum in the form of motivation can be hard to come by, especially if you are mentally and physically exhausted. Figuring out logistics along with finding the necessary energy to exercise can feel overwhelming, which is why most people quit before starting.

Do not choose workouts (or diets, for that matter) based on the latest buzz. Choose workouts where you know you can remain consistent. What good is it to work out seven days this week, three days next week, and not at all for the following three weeks?

It's better to work out three days per week every week for those five weeks, even if it means lowering the intensity to create consistency. This is representative of the story of the tortoise and the hare. It's never about perfection when it comes to health. Remember: consistency over perfection every time.

If you're not exercising at all as a part of your daily/weekly routine, I want you to think about what exercises you tend to like. Everyone has *something* they like to do.

Next, think about what regimen will predict the most consistency based on your preferences.

Finally, how can you set yourself up for success? For some, that could look like enlisting a friend for daily walks. For others, it might mean moving the treadmill up from the dark, lonely basement, and into the family room. Remember, a body in motion stays in motion and a body at rest stays at rest. Choose the former. Choose consistent motion.

choose your plan

Affirmation

Repeat this statement every day this week:

"A body in motion stays in motion."

Action

This exercise is a bit more interactive. Refer to Appendix C if you'd like to give it a try!

Achieve

While choosing organic ensures fewer chemicals and hormones, it's still important to read the food labels to evaluate health and nutrition claims. Start the habit of looking at the nutrition facts panel before automatically placing items into your shopping cart.

Analyze

What are your unique gifts? How will you help others this week using your gift? Write your answers in your journal and commit to them.

Accountability

Answer the below questions in your dedicated healthy lifestyle journal:

What change did you attempt to make this week?

Were you happy with the results?

What challenges did you encounter?

How would you do things differently next time?

5-star recipes

Power Granola

This granola tastes great on its own or as a topping to yogurt and fruit parfaits. It is perfect after a morning workout. This recipe was passed on to me when I taught group weight loss classes at a local hospital, and I have been using it ever since.

Makes 9 (½ cup) servings

Ingredients

2 cups old-fashioned oats
½ cup walnuts
½ cup almonds
½ cup pecans
½ cup flaxseeds
¼ tsp cinnamon
¼ tsp salt
½ cup real maple syrup
½ cup raisins
Low-fat vanilla yogurt (optional)
Fresh berries—blueberries, strawberries, raspberries, blackberries (optional)

Directions

1. Combine oats, all nuts and seeds, cinnamon, salt, syrup, and raisins in a bowl. Mix together until incorporated.
2. Bake for 30 minutes at 300°F on a greased cookie sheet.
3. Serve with yogurt and fruit, or eat alone as a snack. You can also serve this with milk.

Avocado Bean Salad

This is one of Parker's favorite side dishes. He loves flavorful food and is always the first kid in the kitchen to help me cook, which of course, I appreciate so much. This recipe is great anytime, but we tend to use it as a side dish or weekend lunch option. If you're using it for a packed lunch, be aware of the avocado's tendency to brown once cut open.

Makes 8 servings

Ingredients

1 (15 oz.) can garbanzo beans, rinsed and drained
1 (15 oz.) can black beans, rinsed and drained
4 avocados, pitted and chopped
1 cup grape tomatoes, halved
1 cup fresh cilantro, chopped
½ small red onion, diced
½ cup reduced-fat feta cheese
¼ cup lime juice
Salt and black pepper, to taste

Directions

Mix all ingredients in a bowl, season with salt and pepper to taste, and serve.

Source: Adapted from TwoPeasAndTheirPod.com[3]

conclusion

'You Sell Hope'

In more than 15 years of practicing nutrition, the nicest compliment I've ever received from a patient came in 2017.

The patient was originally seeking help in managing pre-diabetes, a clinical diagnosis she had recently received, in addition to wanting to lose a few pounds to put her in a healthier weight range. We quickly hit it off (it felt like I had known her for years) and our appointments enlivened me. She always had a refreshing perspective on her own life and I loved her insight and ability to articulate her feelings. We shared a love for gardening and cooking, making healthy menu planning a shared joy any time she threw a dinner party.

One day, during her appointment, she was a little more serious than normal. She was just diagnosed with cancer. Her initial reaction was to decline chemotherapy and focus on quality of life. It was not my place to offer advice nor was she looking for any. I simply sat there and cried with her.

She had some time to talk more with her family and care team between our appointments and decided to give chemo a shot. We quickly created a plan to maximize nutrient intake and devised a game plan if any side effects manifested.

That is when she looked at me and said, "You sell hope."

It took me by surprise, because I wasn't expecting it, but when I let the weight of her words set in, I realized she had given me a gift. My reaction? I grabbed another couple of tissues, because how do you not cry at something like that? I am happy to report this beautiful lady is thriving two years later!

Look Past Fear, Focus on Hope

"Hope, it is the only thing stronger than fear." These were the words wisely

245

presented by President Snow to Seneca Crane in *The Hunger Games.*[1]

Fear is pretty powerful. Fear has kept me from hiking the Appalachian Trail, because I heard there were snakes out there. Fear has kept me from going back in a hot air balloon, because it turns out I really am afraid of heights. Most of all, fear has kept me from being completely vulnerable in all situations.

I had the opportunity to be interviewed by a friend for a local magazine story on New Year's Resolutions and practical nutrition advice. During the interview, I was asked what got me into nutrition and to share a little of my story. I explained how I was pretty overweight in college, despite starting for a Division II tennis team. My poor eating habits were the culprit.

"Wait, you were fat?!" the interviewer exclaimed. "We need a picture."

"What?! Hold up. I have all these great tips and tools for getting people healthy and you want to focus on how I looked at what was one of the lowest points in my life? I have an image to uphold. I am supposed to be the one with all the answers. What if my patients don't want to see me anymore knowing my history? What if people think I'm a fraud? This feels way too vulnerable and I don't like it!"

She simply laughed and told me my story made me relatable and to stop being so dramatic. If she wasn't a friend of mine, I would have told her to back off, but deep down, I knew she was right.

People don't want an expert talking down on them; they want a friend walking alongside of them. So, I got her a picture and proceeded to want to vomit every time I walked to the mailbox, waiting for the world (rather, our local town), to know my story.

You probably know how this turns out. My friend was right. People actually liked seeing my human side and not an all-knowing machine. My fear of being vulnerable could have stopped me from reaching others and that would have been sad and wrong.

I think about the courage it takes for my patients to come into my office for the first time. I need to give them more credit. A lot of them have fears that need to be validated and rewritten. Fear of failure, fear of judgment, fear of being vulnerable, fear of me knowing their behaviors, fear of exposing their inner voice, fear of getting on the scale, fear of changing their habits, fear of losing their coping mechanisms, fear of giving up their favorite foods, fear of giving up going out to eat or socializing … the list goes on and on.

I joke all the time that the people that walk into my office know what they should be doing, they just have trouble with the execution. Some of that can be taught with tools and tips, but teaching confidence and self-esteem is a completely different challenge to overcome.

Renee Mauborgne stated in an interview, "If I only know where I need to go, but I don't have the confidence to act, I'm not going anywhere."[2]

My closing words are simple: let hope be your courage. Bravery is a choice. It's not an easy choice, but I promise it will take you places you didn't even know existed. My patient gave me a gift that day and now it's time for me to extend that gift to you. I believe in you and can't wait to see what you achieve!

epilogue

Be Good to Each Other, Be Kind to Yourself

A few years ago, I got into the habit of writing out goals for myself the last week in December. I divide my goals into four categories: personal, professional, physical, and spiritual. I write down anything that comes to mind and allow myself to dream big and small. By the time I'm finished, the lists contain somewhere between 30 and 40 items. The whole process makes me giddy and overwhelmed all at the same time.

The first year, I would look at my goal sheets weekly, trying to plan, execute, and check off as many goals as possible. It felt invigorating and the feeling of accomplishment was addicting. I wish I could say I was killing it in the mom/wife role, as well, but that would be a lie. I could only focus on one thing at a time, and checking off boxes was my new favorite hobby.

Sometime in June, I lost my list. I'm pretty sure Jesus was helping me out because He saw I was struggling on the home front. I eventually found the list a few days after Christmas. It was so much fun to read the things I accomplished without even knowing I wrote them down as a goal, that I decided to repeat the practice the following year. As for the things I didn't complete, it was a great opportunity for me to ask myself if that goal was still important enough to write down again.

I'm sure experts would tell you that you should pull out your goals weekly, if not daily, to recommit and stay focused; but, for me, personally, that wasn't working out so well.

I recently watched an interview regarding work-life balance. The interviewee said there was no such thing. You're either killing it with the mom role or killing it professionally, but you can't do both. The interview was meant to be inspiring not defeating, so I'm choosing to look at it that way.

There are days I will be a great mom, but that means my business will take a back seat. Then there will be times I miss my kid's basketball game because I have to go to work. My personal goal is to always minimize missing games as much as possible.

So, we move forward, learning as we go, creating a memory bank of what went well (so we can repeat it) and what didn't work (so we can try a new way). My way of doing things is not *the* way, it's just *a* way. We can all learn from each other—in fact, my greatest source of inspiration, motivation, and ideas are from my patients. Being part of that community is what excites me and drives me to be a better person every day.

I recently was looking at my kids' school pictures, and couldn't help but smile. I feel so fortunate to be a part of all of the amazing, crazy memories each kid brings to our family. Between writing and editing this book, Bella ran into my minivan on her bike and got a concussion; so clearly, the chaos hasn't stopped and isn't going anywhere anytime soon.

I'll leave you with this card my daughter Bella gave my son Ben on his birthday this past year. Rather than making her own card, she recycled the one I had given to her two months prior. I captioned it on Facebook as, "Bella won the award for the most heartfelt card." If you get nothing else from this book, always remember to be good to each other and kind to yourself.

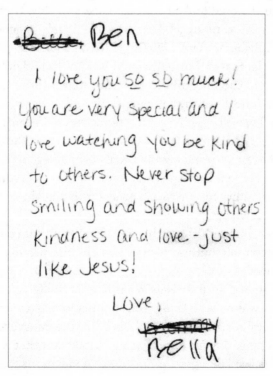

acknowledgements

To Jim—thank you for always being my support and for always making me laugh. I can't imagine doing life without you. I love you!

To Jake—thank you for officially making my dream of becoming a mother a reality. I love your drive and thoughtfulness and I thank Jesus he made me your mom. I love you so much.

To Parker—thank you for continually teaching me how to see people's hearts. I love how you show kindness to others, and I love you so much.

To Ben—thank you for bringing excitement and action to our family. Thank you for providing joy and adventure to our life. I love you so much.

To Charley—thank you for your spunk and adventurous spirit. I love how you make me laugh and I love you so much.

To Bella—thank you for all of your kind notes and encouragement. You are my sweet baby girl and I love you so much.

To my parents—thank you for always believing in me and encouraging me to go after my dreams. I wouldn't be who I am today without your love and support.

To David—thank you for supporting me and all the life lessons you taught me along the way.

To Cathy—thank you for your talent in designing and publishing and listening to me patiently (over and over again) as I tried to explain my vision. Also, thank you for your suggestions with the recipe section.

To Crystal—thank you for all of your creative work in both photographing and designing the front cover. Your eye for creativity, design, and making all things pretty is evident to all who know you. You are super talented and I am so thankful for all of your help!

To my breakfast girls—Carrie, Sara, and Crystal—you are my tribe, my joy, and my greatest fan base. Thank you, thank you, thank you for all of your wisdom, support, love, and encouragement in this project and in life. I can't wait to see what adventures are still in store for us.

To Lauren—thank you for being a great friend and loving my kids even when I can't. Thank you for treating my kids with kindness even when I throw shoes and backpacks on your front lawn.

To Alyssa—thank you for your friendship and for all of our amazing conversations pounding out the miles through our town. Thank you so much for all of your time helping me with both the recipe section and edits. You are one of the busiest people I know, yet you always make time to be there for me (or anyone) when asked. You have been such a great encouragement to me and I value our time together.

To Amy—thank you so much for your time editing the book and making it exactly what I hoped it to be. I am so thankful for your friendship.

To Diane—thank you so much for sacrificing your time on such short notice to make sure the book was ready for print. I appreciate your knowledge, guidance, and support—both with this project and life. Your wisdom is reflected in your teaching and patience, and I'm so grateful for the opportunity to call you my friend.

To Jen—thank you so much for your willingness to jump in and assist with edits, design and encouragement. I am so thankful for all of your flexibility and expertise.

To Kendra—thank you so much for your willingness to help me out at the last minute with editing the book.

To Marie Forleo—thank you for your tag line to all of your videos. Without you, this book would not even be an idea, let alone a real tangible thing of which I am very proud.

To Kevin—thank you for helping me take my thoughts to paper and organizing them in a way that was clear and logical.

To the local fire department—thank you for your patience with me while I was learning to cook.

To the local police department—thank you for always keeping my family safe.

To the staff at BodyMetrix—thank you for all of your hard work and support with both this project and our company. I am so, so grateful for each one of you.

And finally, a huge thank you to my patients—**you** are my constant source of inspiration and motivation. I am so thankful for everything you have taught me and for believing in the work we do at BodyMetrix. It is truly a privilege to walk alongside of you, and I am honored and humbled for the opportunity to do life with you.

appendix a

Meal Plan Template

Grocery List

Produce	Canned Items and Dry Foods	Cleaning Supplies	Dairy Case
_____	_____	_____	_____
_____	_____	_____	_____
_____	_____	_____	_____
_____	_____	_____	_____
_____	_____	_____	_____
_____	_____	_____	_____
_____	_____	**Personal Items**	_____
_____	_____	_____	_____
_____	_____	_____	_____
_____	_____	_____	_____
_____	_____	_____	**Other/Misc.**

Organic	Meats		
_____	_____	**Frozen Foods**	_____
_____	_____	_____	_____
_____	_____	_____	_____
_____	_____	_____	_____
Deli	**Baking Aisle**	_____	_____
_____	_____	_____	_____
_____	_____	_____	_____
_____	_____	_____	_____
_____	_____	_____	_____
_____	_____	_____	_____

Monday _____	Friday _____
Tuesday _____	Saturday _____
Wednesday _____	Sunday _____
Thursday _____	

Download the full-size page at
https://www.bodymetrixpa.com/shopping-list

appendix b

Understanding the Food Label

Serving Size
All the information on the label about calories and nutrients is for one serving. If you eat more than one serving, you get more calories and nutrients.

Calories
Choose foods that help you get the nutrients you need without going over your daily calorie goal. Too many calories leads to weight gain.

Total Fat
For every 100 calories, no more than 3 grams of fat.

Saturated Fat
Less than 10% of total calories should come from saturated fat.

Trans Fat
Limit trans fat to no more than 1 gram per day. If food contains partially hydrogenated oils then it has trans fat. Even if an item has less than half a gram per serving, the label may still say trans fat free.

Sodium
Each day, eat less than 2300 mg of sodium. Aim for less than 250 mg per serving.

Sugar
Aim for less than 5 grams of ADDED sugar per serving. On current food labels, the grams of sugar include both natural and added sugars. This will soon be changing when the new food labels are implemented. Avoid high fructose corn syrup.

Men — 36 grams added sugar per day (9 tsp)
Women — 24 grams added sugar per day (6 tsp)
Children — 12 grams added sugar per day (3 tsp)

Fiber
Look for 3 grams or more per serving. Goal is 25–35 grams per day.

Nutrition Facts

8 servings per container

Serving size   **2/3 cup (55g)**

Amount per serving

Calories   **230**

	% Daily Value*
Total Fat 8g	**10%**
Saturated Fat 1g	**5%**
Trans Fat 0g	
Cholesterol 0mg	**0%**
Sodium 160mg	**7%**
Total Carbohydrate 37g	**13%**
Dietary Fiber 4g	**14%**
Total Sugars 12g	
Includes 10g Added Sugars	**20%**
Protein 3g	
Vitamin D 2mcg	10%
Calcium 260mg	20%
Iron 8mg	45%
Potassium 235mg	6%

* The % Daily Value (DV) tells you how much a nutrient in a serving of food contributes to a daily diet. 2,000 calories a day is used for general nutrition advice.

Download the full-size page at

https://www.bodymetrixpa.com/understanding-food-labels

appendix c

Action:
Find Your Ideal Workout

Answer the following questions below by circling one of the options in order to help you navigate what exercise best suits your preferences and what exercise goals will keep you moving most consistently.

1. I prefer aerobic movement, weight training, or a combination of the two
2. I prefer loud, in-your-face, give-it-all-I-got workouts or quiet, fluid, gentle movement, such as Pilates or yoga
3. I like/dislike sweating
4. I enjoy working out with others or by myself
5. I prefer morning, afternoon, or evening workouts
6. I like to go to a gym or I like to work out at home
7. I can be most consistent working out two, three, four, five, or six days per week
8. I can be most consistent working out for 20 minutes, 30 minutes, 40 minutes, or an hour

Write down the following sentence and prominently display it where you will see it every day:

*"My exercise goal that will yield the most
consistency in my life*

is to _____,
(exercise activity)

for _____,
(exercise duration)

_____.
(number of times per week)

appendix d

5-star recipe index

works cited

Lesson 1. Set Yourself up for Success

1. "The Water in You: Water and the Human Body." USGS.gov. https://water.usgs.gov/edu/propertyyou.html (accessed April 2019).
2. Owings, Justin. "Understanding Bodyweight and Glycogen Depletion." http://justinowings.com/understanding-bodyweight-and-glycogen-de (accessed April 2019).
3. Pollan, Michael. *Cooked*. New York: The Penguin Press, 2013.

Lesson 2. The Practice of Patience

1. Birmingham, Rachael. *Savvy: Ingredients for Success*. Hay House, Inc., 2012.
2. Pollan. *Cooked*.
3. Hockman-Wert, Cathleen; Lind, Mary Beth. *Simply in Season: A World Community Cookbook*. Second Expanded Edition. Scottdale, Pa.: Herald Press, 2009.

Lesson 4. Preparing to Leave Your Comfort Zone

1. Weiss, Liz; Newell Bissex. *No Whine with Dinner*. Manchester: M3 Press, 2011.
2. Wellness Concepts. (well-concepts.com)

Lesson 5. Prioritizing Your Most Precious Gift

1. The Pampered Chef. *It's Good for You—Healthy Recipes for Busy Families*. The Pampered Chef, 2004.

Lesson 6. Body Basics

1. Crosta, Peter. "Viruses: What are they and what do they do?" Medical News Today. https://www.medicalnewstoday.com/articles/279084.php (accessed April 2019).
2. "Clustering of Five Health-Related Behaviors for Chronic Disease Prevention Among Adults, United States, 2013." CDC.gov. https://www.cdc.gov/pcd/issues/2016/16_0054.htm (accessed April 2019).
3. America's Test Kitchen Kids. *The Complete Cookbook for Young Chefs*. Naperville, Ill.: Sourcebooks, 2018.
4. Seinfeld, Jessica. *Food Swings: 125+ Recipes to Enjoy Your Life of Virtue & Vice: A Cookbook*. New York: Random House, 2017.

Lesson 7. Mind-Blowing Lessons You Never Learned in School

1. Salzberg, Sharon. *Real Happiness: The Power of Meditation*. Workman Publishing Company, 2010.
2. Albers, Dr. Susan. Various lectures and speeches. http://eatingmindfully.com/
3. Ray, Rachael. "Super-Size Turkey Meatballs with Spinach and Cheese." Rachael Ray Magazine. https://www.rachaelraymag.com/recipe/super-size-turkey-meatballs-with-spinach-and-cheese (accessed April 2019).

Lesson 8. Do as the Southerners Do

1. Neal DT, Wood W, Labrecque JS, and Lally, P. "How do habits guide behavior? Perceived and actual triggers of habits in daily life." *J Exp Soc Psychol* 48:492–98, 2011.
2. La Flamme, Jena. Various podcasts. https://www.jenalaflamme.com/
3. Ray, Rachael. "Leeky, Creamy Chicken-and-Dumpling Soup." Rachael Ray Magazine. https://www.rachaelraymag.com/recipe/leeky-creamy-chicken-and-dumpling-stoup (accessed April 2019).
4. Homolka, Gina. "Philly Cheesesteak Stuffed Portobello Mushrooms." Skinnytaste.com. https://www.skinnytaste.com/philly-cheesesteak-stuffed-portobello-mushrooms/ (accessed April 2019).

Lesson 9. Keep It Simple

1. "Loneliness Affects Our Immune System." HealthStatus.com. https://www.healthstatus.com/health_blog/depression-stress-anxiety/loneliness-affects-immune-system/ (accessed April 2019).
2. Burton, Dr. Neel. "Our Heirarchy of Needs—True freedom is a luxury of the mind. Find out why." Psychology Today. https://www.psychologytoday.com/us/blog/hide-and-seek/201205/our-hierarchy-needs (accessed April 2019).
3. "Just One-in-Five Employees Take Actual Lunch Break." Right Management. https://www.right.com/wps/wcm/connect/right-us-en/home/thoughtwire/categories/media-center/Just+OneinFive+Employees+Take+Actual+Lunch+Break (accessed April 2019).
4. "Rich and Creamy Tomato Soup." Taste of Home. https://www.tasteofhome.com/recipes/rich-and-creamy-tomato-soup/ (accessed April 2019).
5. Bauer, Elise. "Quick and Easy White Bean Salad." Simply Recipes. https://www.simplyrecipes.com/recipes/quick_and_easy_white_bean_salad/ (accessed April 2019).

Lesson 10. Mind Your Taste Buds

1. MacBride, Elizabeth. "Researchers: You Will Take More Pleasure in Moderation Than Overindulgence." Stanford University. https://neuroscience.stanford.edu/news/researchers-you-will-take-more-pleasure-moderation-overindulgence (accessed April 2019).

Lesson 11. Choosing Happiness

1. Humans of New York, 2013. Facebook. https://www.facebook.com/humansofnewyork/photos/a.102107073196735/519378578136247/?type=3 (accessed April 2019).
2. "Foods That Increase Serotonin: Tryptophan + Carbohydrates." Mental Health Daily. https://mentalhealthdaily.com/2015/04/06/foods-that-increase-serotonin-tryptophan-carbohydrates/ (accessed April 2019).
3. Wellness Concepts. (well-concepts.com)

Lesson 12. It's Time to Set the Record Straight

1. *Lexico, Powered by Oxford, s.v.* "cognitive dissonance," accessed April 2019, https://www.lexico.com/en/definition/cognitive_dissonance
2. Foxen Duke, Isabel. Various webinars and podcasts. https://isabelfoxenduke.com/
3. "How Much Sugar Do You Eat? You May Be Surprised!" New Hampshire Department of Health and Human Services. https://www.dhhs.nh.gov/dphs/nhp/documents/sugar.pdf (accessed April 2019).
4. "balance." *Merriam-Webster.com.* 2011. https://www.merriam-webster.com (accessed April 2019).
5. "moderation." *Merriam-Webster.com.* 2011. https://www.merriam-webster.com (accessed April 2019).
6. Pollan, Michael. *In Defense of Food: An Eater's Manifesto.* New York: The Penguin Press, 2009.
7. Peterson, Kristen. PrimeLifeNutrition.org.

Lesson 13. The Unspeakable Truth

1. "Trends in dietary fiber intake in the United States, 1999-2008." Department of Family Medicine, Medical University of South Carolina. https://www.ncbi.nlm.nih.gov/pubmed/22709768 (accessed April 2019).
2. "Turkey & Black Bean Stuffed Poblano Peppers." Tadych's Econo Foods. https://www.tadychseconofoods.com/recipe/turkey-black-bean-stuffed-poblano-peppers/ (accessed April 2019).

Lesson 14. The Attention Your Body Deserves

1. Leach, Taylor. "Social Media Erupts After 'Vegetarian Fed Chicken Milk' Photo." Dairy Herd. https://www.dairyherd.com/article/social-media-erupts-after-vegetarian-fed-chicken-milk-photo (accessed April 2019).
2. Welsh, Jean A.; Sharma, Dr. Andrea; Abramson, Dr. Jerome L.; et al. "Caloric Sweetener Consumption and Dyslipidemia Among US Adults." JAMA Network. https://jamanetwork.com/journals/jama/fullarticle/185711 (accessed April 2019).
3. "Green Hummus." Super Healthy Kids. https://www.superhealthykids.com/recipes/green-hummus/ (accessed April 2019).
4. Segal, Jenn. "The Best Basic Pesto." Once Upon a Chef. https://www.onceuponachef.com/recipes/basil-walnut-pesto.html (accessed April 2019).

Lesson 15. When Life Gets in the Way

1. "Healthy habits can lengthen life." National Institutes of Health. https://www.nih.gov/news-events/nih-research-matters/healthy-habits-can-lengthen-life (accessed April 2019).

Lesson 16. Know Thyself

1. Mumford, Tracy. "Girls' Life vs. Boys' Life? Magazine covers spark an uproar." MPR News. https://www.mprnews.org/story/2016/09/23/books-girls-life-vs-boys-life-magazine-comparison (accessed April 2019).

Lesson 17. Nurturing and Growth

1. Winfrey, Oprah. *What I know for sure.* New York: Flatiron Books, 2014.
2. Pini, Joseph. "10 Shocking Food Waste Statistics." The Swag. https://www.theswag.com.au/2017/04/20/10-shocking-food-waste-statistics/ (accessed April 2019).

Lesson 18. You are the Master of Your Body

1. McWhorter, John Wesley; Raber, Margaret; Sharma, Dr. Shreela V.; Moore, Laura S.; Hoelscher, Dr. Deanna M. "The Nourish Program: An Innovative Model for Cooking, Gardening, and Clinical Care Skill Enhancement for Dietetics Students." Journal of the Academy of Nutrition Dietetics. https://jandonline.org/article/S2212-2672(17)31928-7/fulltext (accessed April 2019).
2. Paddock, Dr. Catharine. "Soil Bacteria Work In Simiarl Way to Antidepressants." Medical News Today. https://www.medicalnewstoday.com/articles/66840.php (accessed April 2019).
3. "Chickpea, Avocado, & Feta Salad." Two Peas & Their Pod. https://www.twopeasandtheirpod.com/chickpea-avocado-feta-salad/ (accessed April 2019).

Conclusion. 'You Sell Hope'

1. *The Hunger Games.* DVD. Directed by Gary Ross. West Hollywood: Color Force, 2012.
2. Forleo, Marie. "Stop Competing & Start Creating: How to Be Uniquely Successful With Renée Mauborgne." YouTube Video, 28:20. Posted February 2018. https://www.youtube.com/watch?v=YLgUnEtN1Ic